MOTOR CONTROL

Issues and Trends

Contributors

Jack A. Adams
Robert W. Christina
Keith C. Hayes
Steven W. Keele
Raymond M. Klein
Ronald G. Marteniuk
David G. Russell
Richard A. Schmidt
J. A. Scott Kelso
George E. Stelmach
Jeffery J. Summers

MOTOR CONTROL

Issues and Trends

Edited by

George E. Stelmach

Motor Behavior Laboratory and
Department of Physical Education
University of Wisconsin–Madison
Madison, Wisconsin

ACADEMIC PRESS   New York   San Francisco   London   1976

A Subsidiary of Harcourt Brace Jovanovich, Publishers

ACADEMIC PRESS, INC.
111 Fifth Avenue, New York, New York 10003

United Kingdom Edition published by
ACADEMIC PRESS, INC. (LONDON) LTD.
24/28 Oval Road, London NW1

Library of Congress Cataloging in Publication Data

Main entry under title:

Motor control.

Includes bibliographies and index.
1.   Motor learning.   I.   Stelmach, George E.
[DNLM: 1.   Motor activity.   2.   Motor skills.   WE103
M917]
BF295.M66   152.3'34   75-37675
ISBN 0−12−665950−8

PRINTED IN THE UNITED STATES OF AMERICA
80 81 82   9 8 7 6 5 4

Contents

5 The Structure of Motor Programs
Steven W. Keele and Jeffery J. Summers

6 Attention and Movement
Raymond M. Klein

7 Cognitive Information Processes in Motor Short-Term Memory and Movement Production
Ronald G. Marteniuk

8 Proprioception as a Basis of Anticipatory Timing Behavior
Robert W. Christina

9 Dimensions of Motor Task Complexity
Keith C. Hayes and Ronald G. Marteniuk

List of Contributors

Numbers in parentheses indicate the pages on which the authors' contributions begin.

Jack A. Adams (87), Department of Psychology, University of Illinois at Urbana–Champaign, Champaign, Illinois

Robert W. Christina (187), Motor Behavior Laboratory and Department of Physical Education, College of Health, Physical Education, and Recreation, The Pennsylvania State University, University Park, Pennsylvania

Keith C. Hayes (201), Department of Kinesiology, University of Waterloo, Waterloo, Ontario, Canada

Steven W. Keele (109), Department of Psychology, University of Oregon, Eugene, Oregon

Raymond M. Klein (143), Department of Psychology, Dalhousie University, Halifax, Nova Scotia, Canada

Ronald G. Marteniuk (175, 201), Department of Kinesiology, University of Waterloo, Waterloo, Ontario, Canada

David G. Russell (67), Department of Human Movement Studies, University of Queensland, St. Lucia, Brisbane, Queensland, Australia

Richard A. Schmidt (41), Department of Physical Education, University of Southern California, Los Angeles, California

J. A. Scott Kelso* (1), Motor Behavior Laboratory and Department of Physical Education, University of Wisconsin–Madison, Madison, Wisconsin

George E. Stelmach (1), Motor Behavior Laboratory and Department of Physical Education, University of Wisconsin–Madison, Madison, Wisconsin

Jeffery J. Summers† (109), Department of Psychology, University of Oregon, Eugene, Oregon

*Present address: Motor Learning and Performance Laboratory and Department of Physical Education–Men, The University of Iowa, Iowa City, Iowa.

†Present address: Department of Psychology, University of Melbourne, Parkville, Victoria, Australia.

Preface

Motor control is a relatively new endeavor for the behaviorist interested in skilled behavior. Throughout the years, only a handful of experimental psychologists have addressed themselves to motor control. Traditionally, this topic has been in the private domain of the neurophysiologist, but this is no longer so. The behaviorist's interest in motor control can be traced to his fundamental concern for movement accuracy and the variables that underlie it. Until recently, however, the behaviorists made no direct assault on motor control because of the overwhelming influence of S-R associationism theory in experimental psychology. The monopoly of associationism has now been weakened, and emphasis has shifted to the processes intervening between the stimulus and response. With this changing scene, investigators began to perform experiments that utilized behavior techniques that examined such topics as feedback as a regulating agent, the internal representation of sensory information, and the development of a perceptual trace. These efforts quickly demonstrated the benefits of an interdisciplinary approach since it was realized that the neurophysiologist had to relate his findings to behavior. Likewise, the behaviorist realized his need to link his findings to the neuromechanisms that underlie motor control.

This volume addresses nine topics under the general rubric of motor control. Each chapter contains experimental data reflecting current issues and trends. Topics were not selected or intended to be unrelated. The volume was planned for overlap and, hopefully, controversy among authors with the sole concern being that the topics be integrally tied to skill execution. Each chapter briefly orients the reader with background material which is followed by an in-depth treatment of the selected topic, with heavy emphasis on data.

It was not too many years ago that most of skill learning research centered on task-oriented analyses that were so common during the past World War II period. Motor behavior research has moved away from this global approach to skill learning, and now focuses on what has been labeled a process-oriented approach. This volume attempts to evaluate the main ideas which have emerged from this approach.

My intent in developing this book was to bring together a group of scientists who have been doing much of this exciting research and to provide them with a forum to express their ideas. The authors were encouraged not to just review the literature but to take a definite position on many of the issues reviewed based on their own experimental program. In general, most of the authors did this. A second concern was to attempt to provide some unification of a large, diverse, and widely scattered literature in motor control which has often been criticized because of its many disconnected pockets of data. Unification should permit better conceptualization, facilitating theoretical development. Third, the area has changed so rapidly in the last five years that I felt there was a need to put together a volume which covered most of the contemporary issues so that those who have been left behind may have an opportunity to catch up. As such, the book should serve as a basic source and reference for anyone interested in the current issues in motor control.

I would like to thank the authors who have contributed their time and effort, for without their help the completion of the volume would not have been possible. Each of the chapters was reviewed and suggestions made for improvement. I would like to thank all those who helped in the review process: Ann Duncan, Richard Desjardins, Scott Kelso, Peter MacNeilage, Penny McCullagh, Hugh McCracken, and Stephen Wallace.

George E. Stelmach

1

Central and Peripheral
Mechanisms
in Motor Control

J. A. Scott Kelso

George E. Stelmach

I. Introduction

How the central nervous system produces coordinated or patterned motor output is an issue of major concern to those researching the areas of human performance and motor skills. Traditionally, this problem has been food only for the thoughts of physiologists; however, with the ever-narrowing gap between brain and behavior, this is no longer the case. Indeed the multidisciplinary approach to problems of motor control is clearly evident in recent neuroscience publications (Evarts *et al.*, 1971; Massion, 1973; Schmitt and Worden, 1974) and symposia (Teuber, 1974). It seems clear that these reflect a need for a common

1

conceptual level which can be approached by both physiological and psychological data for the development of theory.

In a somewhat similar vein, Schmidt (1975) and Pew (1974) have remarked how the field of motor behavior has shifted only recently, from a global product-performance orientation to one predominantly involved in understanding the processes underlying movement. In vogue with this approach to motor skills and in light of recent theoretical developments (Adams, 1971; Gentile, 1972; Welford, 1972; Whiting, 1972; Pew, 1974) the present chapter attempts to focus on some of the mechanisms involved in motor control. It is not possible to be all-inclusive in this regard. The state of the art permits only the briefest glimpse at what mechanisms may be involved, even in the very simplest of movements. Rather, this chapter will be addressed primarily to the role of the various types of information which may be used by the central nervous system (CNS) in the generation and control of movements. It will be evident, as the chapter unfolds, that considerable disagreement exists; first with regard to what information is actually coded in the CNS, and second, the manner in which the CNS operates on that information. The aim, therefore will be to point out some of the apparent paradoxes which exist in the literature, and, where possible, allude to ways in which they may be resolved. In addition, the empirical base of the chapter will be founded on some recent experiments in our laboratory which focus on the involvement of central and peripheral factors in voluntary movement reproduction. A final aim will be to stimulate ideas and provide possible direction to future research in the area of motor control.

A. Theories of Movement Control

In order to coordinate movement an appropriate set of muscles must be activated in proper temporal relationship to others and an appropriate amount of inhibition has to be delivered to each of the muscles that will oppose the demanded motor act. Historically, two major theoretical attempts have been made to handle these basic requirements, one peripheral in nature and the other stressing central factors. Peripheral control theory clearly recognized the value of sensory information in movement. Coordinated motor output was considered as built up from smaller, discrete phases of movement, linked together by "chain reflexes" with sensory feedback from each phase reflexly initiating each subsequent phase. The cornerstone of this theory was essentially the early experimental work of Mott and Sherrington (1895), who demonstrated the contribution of muscular and cutaneous sensation to purposive movement of a limb in monkeys. When completely deafferented, the limb was virtually paralyzed and grasp was abolished. The findings and more recent replications (Twitchell, 1954; Lassek, 1953) led to the notion that afferent impulses from the skin and muscles (and presumably the joints also) were necessary for the execution of the highest level movement.

Central control theory, on the other hand, claimed that feedback from the movement was unnecessary for the elaboration of motor output. Here it was argued that the higher centers of CNS already possessed the information necessary for movement patterning, and that they did not need to be informed that a particular phase had been completed in order to initiate a further phase. One of the earliest supporters of this position was Lashley, who caused a major theoretical upheaval with regard to how motor sequences were learned and controlled. By severing proprioceptive afferents (Lashley and Ball, 1929) or placing lesions in the rat's cerebellum (Lashley and McCarthy, 1926) no reduction in accuracy of maze running was found, although the outcome of surgical procedures, per se, resulted in motor disturbances sufficient to dramatically alter the motor pattern. These findings, though refuted many times (see Adams, Chapter 4 of this volume) led to a rejection of peripheral "response chaining" theory in favor of the existence of some wholly central mechanism as the determiner of motor sequences (Lashley and Ball, 1929).

Perhaps the primary question relates to how the two theories accommodate the basic requirements of coordinated movement. While the selection of muscles would be met in essentially the same way by both peripheral and central theories, namely, specific neural pathways transmitting impulses to appropriate motoneurons, the temporal and quantitative requirements would have to be met rather differently. Clearly, peripheral control theory could handle these aspects by postulating that afferent activity is fed back to control centers in order to facilitate or inhibit the various phases of movement. Centralists, however, would claim that this method of control was redundant, since the central mechanism already contained the information necessary to specify the temporal and quantitative aspects of the movement.

B. Feedback and Feedforward Concepts

In actual fact when we discuss "response chaining" theory in terms of sensory feedback being responsible for the reflex elicitation of movement, or that central theory assumes an independence of sensory feedback, we are using a term which was not part of either conceptualization of movement control. Although feedback principles have been around for at least 2500 years (see Mayr, 1970, for historical development) the term itself was first coined by Nyquist in 1932 (Cushman, 1958) in his theoretical discussion of methods for improving the linearity and stability of vacuum tube amplifiers. In negative feedback, for example, which has found the widest application, a reference signal (input) and some function of the controlled variable (normally the output) are compared differentially and fed into the amplifier as an error activating signal which can then respond with a corrective signal. Thus, the main characteristic of a feedback control system is its closed-loop structure.

The applications of closed-loop thinking have been immense and are exemplified in the number of theoretical models designed to explain a diversity of processes in many scientific fields. Within the realm of motor behavior, the role of feedback is primarily considered in terms of peripheral information from the various modalities providing the substrate for the detection and correction of movement errors (Adams, 1971; Chase, 1965; Gentile, 1972; Welford, 1972; Whiting, 1972). Adams (1971) is especially explicit in this regard, in proposing that the mechanism responsible for evaluating the correctness of a particular response is developed as a function of the sensory feedback impinging upon it. Thus, the more feedback available, the stronger this mechanism (the perceptual trace) becomes and the more efficient are the processes of error correction and detection. Although proprioceptive feedback was thought to have an equivalent role in developing the strength of the perceptual trace (Adams, 1971), it turns out that this may not be the case. Adams (1972) tested subjects in a linear positioning task under conditions of low and high proprioceptive feedback (added torque on the slide) with vision and audition eliminated. The essential findings were that neither amount of practice nor feedback (both primary constructs in the theory) influenced the detection or correction of errors in performance. Adams' favored interpretation of these data was that he and other closed-loop theorists had erred in accentuating the equality of all feedback channels in error processing. He argued that vision, which was not available in the aforementioned study, may in fact have been the primary determiner of movement accuracy, and has since produced data to confirm this assertion (Adams and Goetz, 1973).

Certainly vision appears to be a dominant modality in strengthening the so-called perceptual trace. Stelmach and Kelso (1975) arrived at such a conclusion using a response biasing paradigm. The question of interest here was whether the effect of an interpolated movement on the recall of a criterion movement could be reduced by providing more feedback during criterion presentation. Subjects made criterion movements with either vision (V), audition (A), heightened proprioception (K), a combination of all three (VAK), or an absence of all three (−VAK), i.e., a blind positioning response. The interpolated movement, which was systematically varied ±40° from the criterion, was always presented in the −VAK mode. Only in the combined feedback and visual conditions was response biasing reduced, further suggesting that Adams (1971) was wrong in equating the input channels in their contribution to trace strength.

Of course, on a number of counts this may not necessarily be the case. First, it might be argued that in neither the Adams (1972) nor the Stelmach and Kelso (1975) studies was proprioceptive feedback properly manipulated. The technique of adding weight to the positioning apparatus seems to have a negligible effect on heightening proprioceptive cues. Recent studies (Christina and Price, 1973; Williams, 1973) using similar methods to increase proprioceptive feedback also failed to demonstrate the effects predicted by Adams' theory. Similarly, Jones (1974a) has criticized the notion put forward by many investigators (e.g., Bahrick, 1957; Gibbs, 1954) that accuracy of lever positioning can be improved by increasing the tension or resistance to movement, on the basis that verbal or visual knowledge of results was always available.

Second, the interpretation that the information channels are differentially important cannot be accepted fully because proprioceptive information was *always* available. Thus, while it is easy to manipulate the role of vision or audition in movement, the proprioceptive modality presents a real problem. Without becoming too involved in this issue at present, it can logically be argued that only by eliminating proprioception can its relative role in regulating the development of the perceptual trace be determined.

Finally, the question must be raised to closed-loop theorists who have predominantly espoused peripheral feedback notions, of whether error processing has anything to do with sensory feedback. With few exceptions (Whiting, 1972) the possible operation of internal feedback loops has been completely ignored in spite of evidence to the contrary (Evarts *et al.*, 1971). Under this system, signals commanding the movement may be compared centrally with the reference mechanism and an appraisal of correctness made without any contribution from peripheral feedback. While we will develop the concept of internal feedback more thoroughly in a later section, two related examples will suffice in pointing out the limitations of the notion that peripheral feedback control is responsible for *all* types of movement.

The first of these is a study by Higgins and Angel (1970), who measured subjects' movement errors in superimposing a cursor on a rapidly moving visual target. A tracking error was defined as any response in which the initial acceleration caused the cursor to move away from the target. Error correction time (ECT) was then defined as the interval between the onset of movement and the onset of deceleration. Comparisons of ECTs with proprioceptive reaction time (PRT) revealed that in all cases mean ECT (range 83–122 msec) was less than mean PRT (range 108–169 msec), suggesting that the subject was able to amend errors without using proprioceptive feedback. Essentially similar findings were reported by Schmidt and Gordon (1974) in a two-choice step tracking task. Schmidt (1975) had earlier argued that the Higgins and Angel (1970) data could easily be explained in terms of the subject producing errors as a result of anticipating the movement direction. Thus the movement could have been preprogrammed but a resulting mismatch between the expected and actual stimuli would lead the subject to initiate a correction. For this hypothesis to be true, the time from the stimulus until the emergence of a corrective movement would be a function of visual reaction time plus peripheral refractoriness. Using a variable foreperiod condition to eliminate anticipation, Schmidt and Gordon (1974) found no evidence of anticipation, yet ECTs were small, sometimes less than 90 msec.

The conclusions from both these studies, while not negating the role of peripheral feedback in other types of motor task, tend to support the idea that subjects can monitor their behavior internally, possibly by comparing the actual motor commands with some internal reference or model for the correct movement. A resulting discrepancy between the actual and intended commands would allow the response to be arrested prematurely, prior to the arrival of peripheral feedback. Thus, while the latter information does not appear necessary for error processing, closed-loop notions of control need not be rejected if it is appreciated that central or internal rather than peripheral feedback is responsible (Adams, 1971, 1972).

In summary, then, it is apparent that closed-loop control systems rely heavily on the concept of feedback and several sources of feedback have been utilized by learning theorists. Clearly, the feedback that is available to the organism will vary depending on its source, the speed of movement required and, to a major degree, the neural substrate responsible for the mediation of feedback. It therefore seems necessary to formally identify the types of feedback which are considered important in the modulation of movement.

    1. Response feedback or information available as a direct consequence of muscular contraction.

    2. External feedback or information available from the environment as an indirect consequence of muscular contraction usually in reference to a goal. Usually referred to as knowledge of results.

    3. Internal feedback or information generated prior to the response from structures within the nervous system.

While we will shortly consider the neural substrate underlying these sources of feedback, let us first discuss briefly the concept of feedforward (McKay, 1966).

It is obvious that the notion of feedforward has not achieved the powerful theoretical status assigned to feedback. Conceivably this may be because it is a less flexible concept than feedback or possibly it may be due to an ignorance on the part of researchers in applying it to motor control problems. It should also be pointed out that in the last 15 to 20 years closed-loop notions have predominated, and feedforward is essentially a form of open-loop control.

Ito (1974) has clarified the notion of feedforward by providing a series of examples in which this form of control is utilized. When a positional change or head movement is signaled by the vestibular apparatus, for example, the vestibulo-ocular reflex will evoke a compensatory movement of the eyes to maintain retinal input constancy. The final output of this reflex will be detected by vision but there is no simple way to return the information to the vestibular organ. Thus, as Ito points out, the vestibulo-ocular reflex operates open-loop in a feedforward manner. Ito further believes, as do many others (Eccles, 1973; Kornhuber, 1974; Pribram, 1971; Allen and Tsukahara, 1974; Teuber, 1974), that feedforward control occurs at higher hierarchical levels in the CNS (Ito, 1970). Thus, the learner's early efforts at movement control would be predominantly dependent on peripheral feedback with higher centers continuously aware of what is being done so that corrections can be made. As learning progresses, however, the large (and slower) external loop to the periphery is no longer indispensable and structures within the central nervous system can take over. Only when an exact "internal model" of desired performance is established (possibly in the neocerebellum) can feedforward control assume the major role. Such an internal model of required performance is not inflexible, but rather can be adjusted from time to time by the various input pathways from peripheral and central sources.

Entirely analogous to the concept of feedforward are notions of efference copy (von Holst, 1954) and corollary discharge (Sperry, 1950; Teuber, 1964). Essentially what is proposed here is that active, voluntary movements involve two sets of signals, both of which operate via feedforward operation: one, the downward discharge to effector organs, and two, a simultaneous central discharge from motor to sensory systems that presets the sensory system for the anticipated consequences of the motor act. We shall have more to discuss regarding this concept from a neurophysiological point of view and when we consider our own data on preselected, voluntary movements. Suffice to point out that internal feedforward control seems a useful theoretical adjunct to closed-loop notions which have stressed the role of peripheral feedback. In fast, "ballistic" movements, for example, feedforward control might be considered the dominant mode, since peripheral feedback cannot be continually processed during the movement execution (Schmidt, 1972). Also, it seems appealing that the human organism shifts as a function of learning from a predominantly feedback mode to a predominantly feedforward mode of motor control. Clearly, there is an element of each type of control at all stages in learning, and neither should be viewed as mutually exclusive of the other. However, it would appear that man does strive to achieve feedforward control, i.e., to preprogram his movements in a highly skilled manner. The empirical data to support a shift in control mode is as yet found wanting. One appealing approach is that of Schmidt and his colleagues (Schmidt, 1969, 1972; Schmidt and Russell, 1972; Schmidt and McCabe, 1972), who have coined the index of preprogramming (IP) as a dependent measure of the extent of feedback utilization in movement. Presumably if the proposed control shift is taking place, less and less use of peripheral feedback should be made as a function of practice and learning. The evidence for this is as yet very tenuous but certainly warrants further investigation, especially in light of the data provided by Adams *et al.* (1972), which rejects the concept that subjects shift to a programming mode as a function of practice.

II. Peripheral Mechanisms
Underlying Movement Control

It is not surprising that, until recently, peripheral control theory has been a dominating influence on those researchers investigating the mechanisms of motor control. When one considers the neurological networks involved in overt motor behavior, it can be found that the majority of such networks are involved in the processing of sensory information (Williams, 1969; Smith, 1969). The fact that a great deal of such input is derived from proprioceptive sources would appear to substantiate the notion that the overt response is considerably influenced by peripheral mechanisms.

Sensory receptors have traditionally been classified on the basis of the information they convey and the manner in which this information is utilized by the central nervous system. Proprioception, for example, can be considered a category of responses from those receptors which are stimulated by actions of the body itself, as opposed to information provided by visual or auditory receptors. The concern for what constitutes man's awareness of his body and limbs and his ability to perceive movement, active or passive, has been the subject of considerable debate for the last 150 years.[1] Bell (1826), for example, considered the muscles to play the primary role, while Duchenne (1883) rejected this notion in favor of the joints. During the early part of this century, however, "muscle sense" (Sherrington, 1906) was considered responsible for the appreciation of limb movement and position.

More recently, as a result of more sophisticated neurophysiological techniques, muscle spindle receptors and Golgi-tendon organs have been excluded since they were thought to be incapable (a) of indicating the absolute length and tension of a muscle necessary for supplying information about limb movement (Boyd, 1954; Mountcastle and Powell, 1959; Merton, 1964) and (b) of accessing central mechanisms (Mountcastle *et al.*, 1952). However, evidence presented by Goodwin *et al.* (1972), Granit (1972, 1973) and others (Eccles, 1973; Sears, 1974) suggest that the role of muscle receptors in providing conscious information of position and movement, should be reconsidered. Furthermore, hypotheses have been developed, which if they can be verified, have important implications for the interaction of central and peripheral factors in motor control (Stein, 1974; Granit, 1972). For this reason we shall consider in the next section the informa-

---

[1] Hopkins (1972) provides a more detailed history of this argument.

tion provided by joint receptors and follow that with a discussion of muscular afferents and their efferent control. Obviously, it would be unwise to consider these peripheral sources of information as separate entities; the accuracy of movement is probably dependent on each, albeit to varying degrees.

A. Joint Receptors

While the contribution of muscle receptors to the perception of position and movement has been the subject of debate in modern neurophysiology, the same cannot be said about joint afferents. The reader is directed to a number of extensive reviews (Skoglund, 1973; Smith, 1969; Howard and Templeton, 1966) which handle the literature adequately; for this reason, the data on the topic will only be considered briefly here.

In analyzing joint afferents from the previously mentioned reviews, the three major types of receptors and their mode of operation are as follows:

1. The Golgi-tendon organs in the ligaments, which are unaffected by the muscles inserting at the joint and thus may signal exact joint position as well as direction.

2. The highly sensitive Ruffini endings which signal speed and direction of movements. Since these are affected by muscle tension at the joints, they may also signal resistance to movement and perhaps discriminate active from passive movement.

3. The Pacinian corpuscles, which may be capable of detecting very small movements as well as movement acceleration (Skoglund, 1973).

The availability of movement and position information provided by peripheral joint receptors consequent on the motor act fits in well with the concept of a closed-loop design. The latter is dependent on faithful transmission of information regarding movement characteristics so that error processing can take place. Presumably, by obtaining knowledge on how joint inputs are coded by higher centers, it should be possible to consider what information is most important to the organism in determining future motor responses. Certainly behavioral investigations on the coding of movement cues (Marteniuk and Roy, 1972; Marteniuk, 1973; Marteniuk et al. 1972) indicate that certain cues are more salient than others for accurate reproduction. The fact that location information is considered primary (Laabs, 1973) would seem to implicate a role for joint receptors, a point explicitly made by Marteniuk and Ryan (1972). They had subjects perform horizontal, straight-arm movements in order to determine the relationship between the physical stimulus continuum and the psychological continuum of kinesthetic extent of arm movement. The linear functions obtained via the methods of fractionation and category production suggested that subjects had a constant sensitivity throughout the movement range, indicating a metathetic or substitutive underlying process (Stevens, 1957). In terms of Skoglund's (1956) classification of joint receptors, it was considered that the Golgi-type endings, which signal exact joint position and presumably act substitutively, were responsible.

While this type of experiment represents a worthwhile attempt at relating the psychophysical properties of the proprioceptive modality to physiological data on joint receptors, it poses two problems of interpretation. First, it seems to assume that receptor firing in the peripheral nervous system in response to a change in limb position [which Skoglund's (1956) data speak to] reflects the coding processes at higher levels of the system. Thus, the subject's subjective responses are interpreted in terms of the firing properties of the receptor, which appears unlikely. Second, the metathetic process proposed by Marteniuk and Ryan (1972) cannot be taken to reflect only the activity of joint receptors, as they conclude. Subjects, for example, after being presented the movement range, moved to where they thought one-ninth, seven-ninths, etc., of the movement would be. In this situation, where the subject actively moves to a self-defined position, motor outflow and muscle receptor sources of information are also likely to be available.

While these studies are informative with regard to the codability of various movement cues, they tell us relatively little about the role of joint afferents in movement control. The type of question which might be asked in this regard might focus on whether we need joint afferents to inform us that we have made a particular movement. Obviously, if we do not, some other source of information must be available for this purpose, at least if we are to subscribe to a closed-loop control model. Clearly, the most direct way to obtain some insight into this problem would be to eliminate joint afferent information. Several studies have attempted to do this by injecting anesthetic into the joint capsule (Browne *et al.*, 1954; Provins, 1958; Goodwin *et al.*, 1972) or by using a blood pressure cuff to render joint sensory nerves anoxic (Merton, 1964; Goodwin *et al.*, 1972). The earlier studies (Browne *et al.*, 1954; Provins, 1958) were concerned with perception of passively induced movement under anesthetic conditions and hence do not concern us here. The experiments of T. Davies, A.J.M. Butt, and P.A. Merton (unpublished, reported in Merton, 1964, 1970) and Goodwin *et al.* (1972), however, had subjects make voluntary finger movements with the cuff inflated at the wrist. By doing this, sensory information below the cuff was effectively eliminated while the muscles mediating finger extension and flexion (since they lie in the forearm) were unaffected. Merton (1964) reported that active movements were made with "much the same accuracy" (p. 394) as under normal conditions; in fact, with similar angular accuracy to eye movements in the dark (Merton, 1961). Similarly, Goodwin *et al.* (1972) had subjects mirror the extension movements of the anoxic finger with the contralateral normal finger. The tracings presented revealed remarkably similar performance in both fingers, with vision, of course, absent.

While the data from these experiments were not quantified in any manner, they do suggest that in voluntary movements joint sense is unimportant. This seems a rather dramatic finding and suggests that other sources of information are available to inform the subject of where and how far he has moved. These presumably could take the form of some internalized information generated within the central nervous system itself, such as "sense of effort" (Merton, 1964), information provided by muscle receptors (Goodwin et al., 1972), or some combination of both. Furthermore, if subjects were programming their responses in a feedforward manner, it would appear necessary to have information about limb position before setting the program into action (Keele, 1973). Nevertheless, according to the data of Davies et al. and the Goodwin et al., prior information about limb position is not available, at least via joint afferents.

Although the above method is open to many manipulations a more thorough investigation of the technique itself is required, as well as the movement characteristics under these conditions. Studies in our laboratory of a similar nerve-block technique applied to the upper arm (Laszlo, 1966) have revealed confounding sensory and motor impairment (Kelso et al., 1974, 1975b). It thus remains to be seen if the "wrist block" used by Goodwin et al. and Davies et al. is void of such factors.

A final, and rather interesting way to examine the role of positional information in movement production might be to consider how location cues are recalled under a variety of presentation modes. The argument here is that if location information (which is likely to be mediated via joint afferents) is the most salient cue for coding movement (Marteniuk and Roy, 1972; Laabs, 1973) the manner in which one moves to the movement endpoint should not differentially affect recall. We performed such an experiment (Stelmach et al., 1975c, experiment 2) in which subjects were asked to reproduce a particular location under preselected (subjects chose their own end point voluntarily), constrained (subjects moved to a stop defined by the experimenter) and passive (subjects were moved to a stop by the experimenter) conditions. Distance information was rendered unreliable by having subjects recall the end point of the criterion movement from different starting positions. The results indicated that the preselected location condition had significantly smaller absolute errors and less variability than the other two conditions. Thus, providing subjects with the opportunity to preselect a particular location prior to movement initiation, which is typically the case in voluntary movement, apparently resulted in superior reproduction.

This finding seems to add further weight to the notion that joint afferents may have a rather limited role in voluntary movements as long as subjects have an accurate "plan" as to where to place their limbs. Thus, as Festinger and Canon (1965) would argue, as long as the subject knows where he wants to move to, no afferent information is necessary to inform him that he has attained that desired position. Efferent information generated within the CNS about spatial location may be sufficient in itself for this purpose. Such a view may be too extreme, however, because there are many situations in which an accurate movement plan is not available. Under these conditions, sensory information from joint receptors may be of paramount importance in informing higher centers of the outcome of the motor act.

B. Muscle Receptors

1. As Feedback Mechanisms

In the conjecture over the role of muscle receptors in serving sensations of position or of limb movement the data provided by Gelfan and Carter (1967) appear to be the most damaging of all. Gelfan and Carter (1967) manipulated under local anesthesia the exposed tendons of patients who were to undergo surgery on the wrist or ankle joint. Although the patients were able to detect applied pressure on the muscle through the skin and connective tissue as well as movement of the joints, they were unable to recognize when the muscle was being stretched by the experimenter pulling on the tendon. It was thus concluded that Sherrington's (1906) "muscle sense" was nonexistent in humans and that there was no conscious perception of the massive influx of neural impulses from the stretch receptors located in muscles.

Though recognizing that this experiment seems at first highly convincing, Granit (1972) rejects the underlying rationale behind it. According to Granit, the spindle component in excitation should not be considered in an isolated manner but only in relation to the associated motor commands that are expressed in alpha-gamma linkage (Granit, 1955, 1970). Thus, since there were no motor commands elicited by subjects in the Gelfan and Carter (1967) experiment, the active exploratory process of perception, in which the spindles are thought to play a role, is excluded. Presumably a similar interpretation can be made of those studies which (a) showed that repetitive stimulation of group 1 muscle afferents in the forelimbs of waking or sleeping cats failed to affect their behavior or desynchronize the electroencephalogram (Giaquinto et al., 1963), and (b) failed to establish conditioned reflexes in cats in response to group 1 stimulation (Swett and Bourassa, 1967; Swett et al., 1964). Hence, just as "meaningless pull on muscles" (Granit, 1972, p. 650) is not regarded as accessing central awareness, so group 1 stimulation isolated from its motor component is unlikely to have any affect.

Contrary to Granit (1972) some recent data suggest that spindles can provide useful proprioceptive information when stimulated in isolation. A series of studies by Goodwin *et al.* (1972) essentially repeated some of the earlier experiments (Merton, 1964; Provins, 1958) which previously had been regarded as cogent evidence against the sentience of the muscle spindle. At the proximal interphalangeal joint of an anesthetized finger, subjects could readily detect movements of $10°-20°$ when they were applied at $5°-10°$ per sec, but had great difficulty in detecting the movement or failed altogether when the velocity was reduced below $1°$ per sec (Provins, 1958). Furthermore, in contrast to Merton (1964), subjects were also capable of detecting movements of below $90°$ in the interphalangeal joint of the thumb after the hand had been rendered anoxic, especially when either the flexors or the extensors were lightly tensed.

These data suggest that the early experiments can be discounted on the basis that they tested the sense of position and movement over relatively small movement ranges and at low movement rates; that is, below the sensory threshold for muscle afferent information. Clearly, this is much higher than that for joint afferents, although no psychophysical scaling (Marteniuk and Ryan, 1972; Hoff, 1971; Ronco, 1963) has yet been attempted. The major point here, however, is that muscle receptors do contribute to conscious proprioception. This fact is perhaps brought out most potently in a very recent study by Matthews and Simmonds (1974) which essentially replicated the earlier investigation of Gelfan and Carter (1967), with rather different results.

In the Matthews and Simmonds study the finger flexor tendons at the wrist were exposed under local anesthesia in five patients who were receiving treatment for "carpal tunnel syndrome." The hand was stabilized while the tendon studied was pulled to and fro with fine forceps (5 mm at 2 Hz) so as to stretch the muscle without moving the relevant digit. Without exception, subjects were able to report when the finger was being moved and when it was immobile. This "illusory movement" produced by pulling the tendon was approximately matched by a real movement of between $5°$ and $10°$ at the proximal interphalangeal joint. Contrary to Gelfan and Carter (1967), these data suggest that afferent discharges elicited by muscle stretch are perceived as movement sensations. The discrepancy between the studies may be attributed to the manner in which the subjects were asked to describe their sensations. Gelfan and Carter (1967), for example, asked their subjects about sensations referable to the muscles, while Matthews and Simmonds (1974) focused their subjects' attention on sensations referable to finger movement. In neither study, however, was an exhaustive analysis of the subjects' sensations made. As De Jong (1951) has emphasized, subjects undergoing neurological testing are highly susceptible to the suggestibility of the experimenter. However, in favor of the Matthews and Simmonds (1974) study in this regard is the finding that subjects did not report movement sensations when the tendons were vibrated at 100 Hz. This would have been expected had subjects been conforming to the anticipations of the experimenter.

While these studies provide evidence of the role of muscle afferents in providing useful feedback information, they await physiological verification. Unlike the various joint receptors, the individual contribution of each of the muscle afferents (primary and secondary endings, Golgi-tendon organs) is not easily assessed. It might be speculated that rapid movements, which are readily detected after paralysis of joint afferents, might indicate a major role for the primary spindle ending which is extremely sensitive to dynamic stimuli. Although their data are hardly convincing, Paillard and Brouchon (1968, 1974) support this notion. They had subjects estimate with one hand the position of the other which was either actively or passively moved to a target. The results revealed that estimation of the actively positioned target hand was significantly more accurate than the passively positioned. The authors concluded that while joint receptors probably acted similarly under active and passive movement conditions, activity of spindle receptors was certainly different and could have been responsible for differences.

This speculation is unwarranted since other sources of information, both peripheral and central in nature, are as likely to have a role in the superiority of active versus passive movement. Skoglund (1973), for example, reviews data which show that receptors of the joint capsule are influenced by muscular action at a joint (Eklund and Skoglund, 1960), suggesting that the pattern and frequency of joint receptor discharge differ under active and passive conditions. Also the availability of internal signals derived from the efferent patterns of motor commands could account for active movement superiority, since these are not present under passive conditions. Finally it might be asked of the Paillard and Brouchon (1968, 1974) studies in which one part of the body is used to locate .its paired member, just *what* is being measured: the position sense accuracy of the reference limb; the accuracy of similar mechanisms in the opposite limb; or the effectiveness with which sensations of one limb can be equated with those of the contralateral limb? Clearly these methodological and logical problems do not aid in clarifying the relative roles of joint and muscle inputs in providing usable proprioceptive information.

The bulk of the physiological and psychological evidence seems to support the greater importance of joint receptors for the encoding of movement (Skoglund, 1956, 1973; Marteniuk et al., 1972). Their well-established cortical representation (Mountcastle and Powell, 1959; Rose and Mountcastle, 1959), compared to the apparent diffuseness of muscular afferent projections (Oscarsson, 1967; Matthews, 1972), is in congruence with this notion. There are, however, conditions in which joint information appears to be overridden by muscle information for processing by higher centers in the central nervous system. It is these situations which may clarify the role of receptors in muscle, not as limited sources of proprioceptive feedback, but as important elements in human movement control.

2. In Efferent Control

One indicant of the role of muscle receptors in motor control is suggested in experiments by Hollingworth (1909) in which constant errors at recall were directly related to the force of impact at a stop which defined the standard movement. Granit (1972) interprets this result in terms of an isotonic contraction being suddenly made isometric. As a result of hitting the stop, spindle discharge would be increased, hence facilitating the motoneurons which in turn would respond to supraspinal commands by increasing their output. The fact that the position of the limb does not change as a result of hitting the stop, yet gross constant errors occur, suggests that muscle afferent excitation overides the "veridical" information provided by joint receptors. If this is what is happening, it indicates that the state of muscle receptor firing following a criterion response determines to some degree the accuracy of the estimation.

One of our experiments speaks to this issue (Stelmach et al., 1975c, experiment 2). We had movement conditions in which subjects moved actively or were moved passively into a stop at a rapid rate, to define the criterion movement. We also had a "nonstopped" condition in which subjects were allowed to define their own criterion. Recall was either immediate or after 15 sec. On the basis of Granit's interpretation of Hollingworth's experiment, it might have been predicted that greater positive constant error would be evidenced in the stopped relative to the nonstopped condition. However, there were no significant differences in constant error among the three movement conditions, which also behaved similarly along the dimension of extent. Thus, in a reproduction paradigm where the subject returns to the starting position after the criterion movement the effect of impact appears to be minimal in terms of biasing the recall response. Ideally, however, it would be interesting to examine the spindle response by employing Vallbo's technique (Hagbarth and Vallbo, 1968; Vallbo, 1971, 1973) of recording directly from human muscle spindles.

A second situation, in which joint receptors fail to record accurately limb movement and position, occurs when vibration, which acts primarily by exciting the large spindle afferents, is applied to the biceps muscle. Experiments by Goodwin et al. (1972) and McCloskey (1973) revealed that when the vibrated arm was prevented from flexing, subjects experienced a feeling of extension, though none could actually occur. When subjects were instructed to track the vibrating events with the contralateral arm, they responded with an extension. Thus, once again muscle afferent information was processed at higher levels leading to illusions of movement similar to those found in the Matthews and Simmonds (1974) study.

How does one interpret these illusory affects which seem to arise as a result of inducing abnormal afferent discharge from muscle receptors? Consider the ways in which the central nervous system might use the information it receives via muscle afferents. For example, on commanding a movement, higher motor centers could be continuously informed about its progress so that corrections could be applied if the actual movement differed from the one commanded. Thus, the movement could be controlled by continuously comparing the actual with the expected performance and the difference used for the purpose of initiating corrective action. While such a comparison process might take place efficiently in a reflex manner at spinal cord level [in the manner of the follow-up servo proposed by Merton (1953)], it would also seem important that higher centers should be involved, since they are more directly related to the commanding of movement. This in fact is Granit's thesis (1972, 1973), where it is argued that the known projections of spindle afferents to the sensorimotor cortex (Oscarsson, 1965; Andersson *et al.*, 1966) form part of a mechanism for checking the execution of movements in relation to motor commands. That muscle spindles can be activated from the cortex (Granit, 1970, for review) and that voluntary acts are characterized by the coactivation of extrafusal (main muscle) and intrafusal (spindle) muscle fibers (Hagbarth and Vallbo, 1968; Vallbo, 1971, 1973) suggest that the spindles are a unique end organ reflecting both demand and execution. Thus, the demanded act is expressed in alpha-gamma linkage to the muscles and its accomplishment is checked by information returning to the cortex. Typically, this checking process is viewed as automatic; hence, when the movement is carried out as planned, afferent information from muscles will not protrude into consciousness unless a mismatch occurs between expected and received information.

Consider the previously discussed illusion findings of Goodwin *et al.* (1972), where the vibrated muscle was perceived as being more stretched than it actually was. When the vibrated arm was prevented from flexing by an external restraint, this was experienced as a feeling of extension, presumably because of the mismatch entailed between what was expected and the feedback to the cortex of group 1A afferent information from the spindles. Only the unexpected was perceived with the vividness to give an illusion. As Eccles (1973) elucidates on the Granit (1972) hypothesis: "Quite a lot of the 1A input to cerebrum isn't appreciated normally, but, when it is disordered, when there is some mismatch as in the illusions, then you know that it's getting through to consciousness [p. 120]." The test of this hypothesis seems at first glance theoretically clear. If receptors other than those in the muscle were anesthetized, e.g., by an inflated cuff around the wrist which would not affect relevant finger flexor-extensor muscles lying in the forearm, and the blindfolded subject was asked to make a voluntary displacement interrupted by an experimenter-defined stop, he should be able to perceive that the movement has been obstructed on the basis of muscular information. Thus, a planned displacement has been "perturbed" unexpectedly and a mismatch should access central awareness. Early unpublished experiments by T. Davies *et al.* (Merton, 1964) revealed that in fact subjects could not perceive when the movement was obstructed after joint receptors had been rendered insentient. Similarly Brindley and Merton (1960), in their study of eye movements under local anesthesia, found that the subject was unable to detect when a voluntary eye movement was prevented from taking place by the experimenter's forceps. These findings would tend to negate the Granit (1972) hypothesis that muscle afferents provide a central checking mechanism for voluntary movements, since subjects should have been aware when their movement plan was not carried out.

The problem, however, with rejecting Granit's (1972) proposal on the basis of the above results is that Goodwin *et al.* (1972) have essentially repeated the Davies *et al.* experiment, using the same technique with entirely opposite findings! Subjects could readily detect randomly placed obstructions, presumably on the basis of an alteration in muscle afferent firing. The reason for the dichotomous result was probably due to the earlier experiment using a rather smaller range of movement, apparently about 20°. However, if the mismatch between the motor commands and the spindle afferent discharge occurs only with larger movements as Goodwin *et al.* (1972) imply, it does not say much for the potency of muscle feedback mechanisms, per se, in closed-loop motor control.

Before reaching any concrete conclusion on this issue, there are a number of points which might be raised. One is that the nature of the "mismatch" has yet to be quantified in a meaningful manner. If we assume on the basis of the Goodwin *et al.* data that subjects can perceive an obstruction in the presumed absence of joint afferents, how accurately can they reproduce the end point at which the obstruction occurred? This would allow us to understand what the hypothesized "mismatch" is actually doing; whether it is merely informing the subject that an obstacle has occurred "somewhere" in the path of movement or whether it can provide information about the actual position of the obstacle. Also, what is the role of corollary discharges (Teuber, 1964; Sperry, 1950) which are thought to accompany voluntary movements by presetting sensory systems for the anticipated consequences of the motor act? The early experiments on subjects with anoxic hands who perceived voluntary movements whether or not the thumb was obstructed by the experimenter (Merton, 1964) fitted well into this idea. However, the Goodwin *et al.* (1972) study favors the muscle afferent interpretation. Clearly this issue has to be resolved before any progress can be made. A principal question, to which we will not turn, surrounds the information which corollary discharge may provide (a point also of concern to Adams; see Chapter 4, this volume) relative to that obtainable from muscle receptors.

3. Relationship to Corollary Discharges

The beauty of the original follow-up servo theory of spindle control (Merton, 1953), as pointed out by Matthews (1974), was that it did not matter to the nervous system whether spindle discharges were elicited by passive stretch of the main muscle or by gamma activity initiated centrally. In both cases the end result was the same; namely, the discharge of alpha motoneurons and resultant muscle contraction.

Recent studies, however (Marsden *et al.*, 1972, 1973; Merton, 1974; Evarts, 1973; Evarts and Tanji, 1974), indicate that muscular afferents access cortical structures in what has been termed a transcortical or long loop reflex (Phillips, 1969). Marsden *et al.*, for example, investigated the response produced by various conditions of loading and unloading muscle spindles during constant velocity flexion movements of the top joint of the thumb. The electromyogram (EMG) response to unexpectedly presented perturbations was a reduction when the movement was allowed to accelerate, an increase when it was halted and a further increase when the movement was reversed. However, the response latency under all conditions was similar (approximately 50 msec), indicating that this response was equivalent to the load-compensation servo action predicted to occur with alpha-gamma coactivation (Granit, 1970); that is, an automatic attempt to compensate for the perturbations by reflexly turning the muscles on or off. The long latency involved, which is more than twice as long as spinal reflex time, has led to the notion that the stretch reflex and servo action may have been taken over by the cerebral cortex.

The implications of these findings, and similar ones by Evarts (1973) with monkeys, are that it must matter to higher centers whether the afferent firing was evoked by muscle stretch or by gamma motor activity. This problem can be solved, at least theoretically, if higher centers are informed of the extent of motoneuronal firing as well as receiving afferent information. This would necessarily implicate a "copy of command" or corollary discharge, with which returning afferent signals could be compared and a mismatch computed. The nature of this interaction and the level at which it takes place is probably the most intriguing question to those researchers interested in motor control.

Granit (1972) however, has rejected the concept of corollary discharge, apart from the gamma loop through the spindle and back to the sensorimotor cortex. This view seems somewhat short-sighted, since by accepting the notion that muscle afferents contribute to kinesthesia (as Granit does), it would seem necessary to implicate corollary discharges. This is so because "raw" afferent signals from muscles have no absolute meaning in themselves, except in relation to the degree of motor activity. Thus, for any meaning to be extracted from spindle input it would seem important that some comparison between the information expected on the basis of the planned movement and the actual sensory consequences of the movement executed should be made.

The question of whether corollary discharge, in and of itself, can contribute to conscious perception of movement without the additional aid of afferent input to interact with it, has been a difficult one to answer. One experiment by Goodwin *et al.* (1972) and reported further by Matthews (1974) suggests that it does not. Subjects were instructed to make finger extension movements at various times throughout the duration of a compression block (cuff) applied above the elbow. Their task was to mirror the finger movements of the "cuff" limb with the same finger (index) of the normal, "uncuffed" hand. After about 25 min, subjects were still making movements under "cuff" conditions but apparently were unable to perceive them, reflected by the finding that they made no movements with the normal limb. The point here is that if corollary discharges were mediating some "sensations of innervation" (von Helmholtz, 1867) the subject should have continued signaling the occurrence of a movement. The opposite finding suggests that corollary discharge, in the absence of returning afferent input, cannot give rise to sensation.

Perhaps this conclusion should be treated with some caution, since subjects progressively underestimated the movements made with the cuffed limb. This suggests the possibility that subjects could have recognized on the basis of afferent feedback that progressive paralysis was taking place. However, once the cuff was shifted to the wrist, allowing muscle afferents to recover but maintaining joint afferents insentient, the subject was apparently able to estimate the movements quite well. This finding indicates once again that muscle afferents can provide the necessary movement information to the subject even with joint afferents nonoperational.

The logical inference from the results of these studies suggests a number of future experiments. If indeed joint afferents are of little use under voluntary conditions where the subject knows the movements he wishes to produce, as Merton (1964, 1970) and Goodwin et al. (1972) suggest, we are left with only two sources of movement information: muscle afferents and corollary discharge. The problem would then be to experimentally eliminate one source or the other. An obvious way to eliminate the influence of corollary discharge would be to utilize passive movements where no motor outflow is elicited. However, as indicated earlier, muscular afferent signals must also be interpreted in relation to motor commands. Thus, to assess the relative importance of both muscular afferents and corollary discharge, these sources would have to be manipulated in an active movement paradigm. The alternative approach would be to attempt to remove spindle influences via a gamma motoneuron block (Rushworth, 1960). The problems of infiltrating an anesthetic drug into the fusimotor system are well known (Shambes, 1969; Smith et al., 1972) but the absence of knowledge in this area of human motor control warrants a further effort. The rewards of such an approach, which has been suggested a number of times (e.g., Paillard and Brouchon, 1968; Phillips, 1971), are readily apparent. By selectively removing spindle support, the role of the central command system may be more fully assessed. A suggested design might focus on the accuracy of voluntary movement with and without muscle spindle influences. No differences in movement duplication would reflect the importance of the corollary discharge notion and reduce the presumed role of the spindle (Granit, 1972). Differences between the conditions would reflect the importance of the spindle in volitional motor control.

Throughout the foregoing discussion, the concept of corollary discharge has been alluded to quite frequently. That this has been necessary is of course a reflection on the approach which has been adopted, but it also points to the difficulty in considering peripheral and central processes as mutually exclusive of each other. Nevertheless, there are data (Delong, 1971; Schmitt and Worden, 1974) indicating that under certain circumstances movement sequences can be carried out regardless of afferent information concerning the initial conditions or progress of the movement. Let us now turn to a brief consideration of these findings and also some of the neurophysiological research directed at elucidating the possible mechanisms involved. The reader is directed to Evarts (1971a) for a more complete, though possibly less critical, approach to these data.

III. Central Mechanisms Underlying Movement Control

Evidence for central motor control comes from a number of sources. In an attempt to provide a coherent presentation the data will be dichotomized into two categories, neither of which should be considered exclusive of the other. The first refers to research which has adopted a neurophysiological approach, including (1) studies on endogenous neural networks that elicit patterned motor output independent of peripheral feedback; (2) studies which have manipulated sensory feedback via deafferentation or temporary nerve block; and (3) studies which have attempted to elucidate upon so-called central feedback loops which operate prior to movement. A typical procedure in the latter has been to record the response of single cells during conditioned movements in structures hypothesized to be involved in the monitoring of motor output, as opposed to the more classical approach of studying structures involved in the processing of sensory input.

A second category of studies from the behavioral domain have implicated central mechanisms and include (a) clinical studies of perceptual deficits following frontal lobe lesions; (b) studies which point to the importance of active, self-produced movement for perceptual adaptation; and (c) studies in which sensory feedback, although present, is not considered to be effective in motor control. Examples of the latter are the classical work on voluntary eye movements (von Helmholtz, 1867; von Holst, 1954; Brindley and Merton, 1960), the analysis of performance in so-called "ballistic" tasks, already alluded to in an earlier section, and, finally, the investigation of reproduction accuracy in voluntary versus constrained and passive movements. Clearly, it is beyond the scope of this chapter to deal with all the evidence in the foregoing classification in anything but a representative manner. An effort will be made, however, to provide an understanding of the manner in which central mechanisms have been investigated. In addition possible alternative interpretations for some of the data will be presented.

A. Neurophysiological Research

1. Central Programming

One of the most interesting examples of a centrally elicited pattern of muscle contractions which is independent of the stimulus used to evoke the response is the act of swallowing in mammals. Attempts to alter the pattern by interrupting feedback loops via excision of participating muscles, for example, fail to bring about any significant change in the movement pattern (Doty, 1968). Additional evidence of more complex patterned output in the absence of peripheral feedback is provided by studies on bird song development, recently alluded to by Keele (1973). Konishi (1965), for example, deafened young birds after exposure to adult birdsong and found no deficit in the song pattern the following spring. On the other hand, young birds not exposed to adult song prior to deafening failed to develop a copy of the adult song.

These findings might be explained in terms of Marler's (1970) theory where it is postulated that in learning a bird song, an acoustic memory or "template" of the adult song pattern is formed. The motor output is then compared with the stored reference template and gradually molded to it. Once normal song is acquired, the auditory template is no longer required since the motor output has become centrally organized or programmed and is no longer dependent on peripheral feedback. The neurophysiological mechanisms by which the initial comparison and eventual shift to central programming take place have not been elucidated. Additionally, these data on birdsong indicate an early role for peripheral feedback in the establishment of the central program.

That sensory feedback is not necessarily required at initial learning stages, however, is suggested by a recent deafferentation study on monkeys (Taub et al., 1973). In earlier research, Taub and Berman (1968) had found, contrary to the previously cited findings (Mott and Sherrington, 1895; Lassek, 1953; Twitchell, 1954), that following both unilateral and bilateral forelimb deafferentation, monkeys are able to use their limbs adaptively in conditioning experiments and in locomotion. The problem with Taub and Berman's (1968) studies is that vision, which has been shown to be very important in the recovery of extension and grasp in a deafferented limb (Bossom and Ommaya, 1968; Vierck, 1971; Bossom, 1974), was almost always present. Obviously this source of sensory information could have been responsible for the laying down of movement memory traces. However, by blinding and deafferenting neonate monkeys, Taub *et al.* (1973) found that accurate and coordinated movements were still possible (e.g., using forearms for support, clasping objects, walking), presumably controlled by autonomous central processes. Just how the central processes allow the animals to know first of all to grasp, and then what to grasp remains obscure (Bossom, 1974).

A recent experiment by Levine and Ommaya (1974) raises the same type of question, and allows us tentatively to posit an alternative interpretation to the centralist notion. In this study, monkeys with bilateral rhizotomy were trained to squeeze a rubber bulb taped into one hand in order to obtain a juice reward. Animals were rewarded or not depending on their ability to output and maintain the required pressure. In spite of the absence of feedback graded in terms of muscle contraction, the deafferented monkeys produced very accurately controlled finger pressure as well as normal monkeys. At first glance, this result seems impressive in terms of the precision of control possible in the presumed absence of proprioception. The question to ask, however, to this and earlier deafferentation studies is: Could any other course of information have mediated the observed performance? If, for example, finger muscle output was tightly coupled with some other action such as jaw muscle contraction (e.g., gritting the teeth), the animal could have gauged his effort on the basis of proprioceptive feedback from this activity (Frank, reported in Granit and Burke, 1973). As Bossom (1974) points out, such an interpretation is not far-fetched, since ". . . monkeys are quite capable of such subterfuges, and suitable controls for them have not been generally incorporated into some of the behavioral tasks which have been used [p. 294]."

The foregoing notion is rather interesting in light of some recent work in our laboratory using the nerve compression block to reversibly "deafferent" human subjects (Laszlo, 1966). A common observation when subjects were attempting to perform a tapping task under these conditions was that of extraneous movements, ranging from excessive shoulder rotation to nodding of the head and foot tapping (Kelso, 1973). While such "nonspecific" motor behavior has not been discussed in earlier studies (Laszlo, 1967a,b; Laszlo *et al.*, 1969), its presence limits to some degree the interpretation that motor learning occurred as a result of an internal feedback loop capable of monitoring its own neural impulses without peripheral influences (Laszlo and Bairstow, 1971). Rather it remains a possibility that ". . . remaining pathways to the central interpreter suffice to throw sentient circuits into action [Granit, 1973]," thus reflecting the neural plasticity of the central nervous system in overcoming deficiencies of sensory input.[2]

---

[2] Some may argue that the subject could centrally monitor the efferent impulses for extraneous movements in order to mediate performance. The issue, however, is whether other sensory sources are available for this purpose.

In any case there are genuine problems in accepting the nerve compression block data of Laszlo and her colleagues as evidence for central control, which a number of investigators seem to have done (Docherty, 1973; Keele, 1974; Pew, 1974; Jones, 1974b). In one of our studies (Kelso *et al.*, 1974) negligible tapping performance was found in most subjects in spite of eight sessions designed to allow for improvement. In addition, progressive reduction in motor nerve conduction parameters (nerve conduction velocity and muscle action potential amplitude) occurred across and below the block with significant decrements as early as 15 min. These data, and those of a consequent study (Kelso *et al.*, 1975b) indicated that motor impairment was a confounding factor in the use of the nerve block technique. Finally, recent data of Coggeshall *et al.* (1973) revealing the presence of unmyelinated sensory fibers in ventral (motor) roots may also be significant in light of theory developed from deafferentation studies. The implication here is that such fibers may possibly mediate proprioception in spite of the dorsal root transection traditionally undertaken to remove proprioceptive influences. While it remains to be seen whether this is true or not the suggestion alone tends to reduce the impact of postulated central mechanisms.

2. The Internal Feedback Loop

In spite of reservations in accepting the deafferentation data as unmitigated evidence for central control, there are some neurophysiological data which suggest the presence of internal feedback mechanisms. As Evarts (1973) has pointed out, the discovery that precentral (motor) cortex, basal ganglia, and cerebellum all discharge prior to movement led to a new notion of the functional relationship between the three structures and the implication of an internal feedback loop. How this loop operates in relation to movement and what its exact role is in control remain somewhat speculative.

The crucial question usually asked in the neurophysiological investigation of internal feedback is: Do modifications of discharge occur prior to movement as a result of inputs from other CNS structures, or do they occur following movement, presumably as a result of sensory feedback from the periphery? For example, the concept of corollary discharge as defined earlier implies a neural response in sensory systems before the arrival of response-produced feedback. Clearly, "sensory" systems can be defined at various levels in the CNS including the cerebellum, the thalamus, and the postcentral (sensory) cortex itself. Thach (1970a,b), for example, had monkeys move a lever as quickly as possible in response to visual input and found that cerebellar neurons changed frequency not only after movement but also before it occurred. Early changes of 80–100 msec before any observed change in arm or trunk EMG or force on the lever eliminated the possibility of feedback intervention from the movement and seem likely to have been related to the motor commands. Evarts (1971b), using a similar pardigm, recorded from neurons in nucleus ventralis lateralis (VL) of the thalamus as well as the motor cortex (MC). Activity in VL neurons, like that of the cerebellum, preceded response onset within a 10–110 msec range, suggesting a role for VL neurons in controlling MC activity prior to movement.

Based on the foregoing findings that cerebellar and thalamic neurons are active in advance of movement, Evarts (1972a,b) has asked the question of whether neurons in the sensory cortex also discharge prior to movement via a cerebello-thalamo-cortical input. Although the earliest postcentral discharges occurred 10–40 msec prior to the EMG response, it was not clear whether these were related to feedback from the periphery or to central inputs.

While the foregoing research by Evarts and Thach suggests the operation of internal feedback mechanisms, the present state of the art does not allow for unequivocal acceptance. Methodological factors, seldom discussed in review articles (e.g., Evarts, 1971a), must also be considered. Evarts (1971b), for example, could find only with great difficulty a very small proportion of VL neurons related to the actual movement; "even when all misdirected penetrations are eliminated it remains a fact that units related to the movement were hard to find, even though the electrode was advanced during task performance [p. 324]." Furthermore, one of the major problems in the Evarts' (1972a) study was determining to which muscle the activity of a single motor cortex neuron should be related. It was not possible to establish whether, in fact, it was the hand and finger muscles to which motor cortex cells were related as opposed to other muscles whose discharge was correlated with hand and finger muscles (Evarts, 1972a). Because this was not known, the interval between the onset of activity change in central neurons and the first muscular response could not be determined.

This type of problem in neurophysiological research prompted Llinas (1974) to point out that in order to establish a causal relationship between unitary responses and behavioral events a high correlation between the two must be found. This in itself is probably an oversimplification, since a particular motor performance involves the activation of many neuronal circuits making a precise correlation unlikely. Without wishing to belabor the point, the implications for the investigation of internal feedback loops are rather clear; the operations of postulated central mechanisms must be tightly coupled to the performance generated, otherwise the inferences made are at best tenuous.

3. Cerebro-Cerebellar Connections

Probably the most established evidence for internal feedback comes from the investigation of cerebro-cerebellar connections and their functional significance (for reviews, see Evarts and Thach, 1969; Allen and Tsukahara, 1974). These data may allow us to provide a neurophysiological response to some of the criticisms typically made of internal feedback notions, such as efference copy or corollary discharge.

One of the common criticisms relates to the comparison process between the copy of the command to the muscles and the sensory feedback from the limbs. Since the former is in code for causing muscle contractions, i.e., an output code, and the latter is in a peripheral, or input code, how can they ever match? Without going into the neuronal circuitry involved, the cerebellum is known to receive inputs from both cortical and sensory sources. Furthermore, it can adjust its output on the basis of these inputs (Thach, 1972; Oscarsson, 1972) thus making it an eminent possibility that it can perform a comparative function. There is therefore no reason why the requirement of extensive recoding of central and peripheral inputs should be cited against the notion of efference copy, since the integrational machinery (Eccles, 1973) of the cerebellum seems perfectly equipped for the job.

A more damaging criticism focuses on the type of information that efference copy can provide to the performer. It has been argued that the match of efference copy with incoming sensory feedback can only inform the subject that the movement commanded was carried out as planned, but not about the correctness of the movement with respect to the desired outcome. Thus, efference copy relays information of the extent to which the movement plan was carried out, and not whether the plan itself was appropriate.

This problem can be rather easily handled if one ascribes to Eccles' hypothesis of dynamic loop control (Eccles et al., 1967), which is receiving increasing support as a model of cerebro-cerebellar function (e.g., Allen and Tsukahara, 1974). In this hypothesis, the cerebellum is presumed to carry an immense store of information coded in its specific neuronal connectivities (see Marr, 1969, for a theory on how this may take place). Thus, in response to a pattern of pyramidal tract discharge (representing the motor command), the cerebellar nuclei can compute its "correctness" and return the appropriate modification to the same area of the cerebrum. In this way the accuracy of the movement plan can be checked prior to the influence of peripheral feedback, an internal loop time estimated to be one-fiftieth of a second (Eccles, 1973, p. 130). The longer feedback loop from the periphery relaying the actual sensory consequences could then be sufficient, in itself, to inform higher centers whether the planned movement was executed properly.

Furthermore, some recent Russian experiments cited by Oscarsson (1972) indicate that ascending pathways to the cerebellum are involved in signaling events within the nervous system rather than the periphery. Locomotion was investigated in mesencephalic cats and correlated with the activity of central neurons without the need for anesthesia. While deafferentation of a hindlimb had little effect on the locomotor pattern, it did result in the abolition of rhythmic discharge in sensory neurons traveling to the cerebellum via the dorsal tract. However, ventral tract neurons continued to discharge at predeafferentation level, indicating that their activity was related more to the descending command signals at the segmental level rather than peripheral feedback. This suggests that an internal feedback loop can assess the nature of the planned movement by relaying the effects which the command signals have evoked in lower motor centers back to the cerebellum, which in turn can modify further cortical outputs.

In conclusion, perhaps the most interesting aspect of the internal loop notion is the enhanced theoretical status proposed for the concept of feedback as the major determiner of motor responses. Thus, when it is reported that the motor program is "... based upon the inability of feedback control mechanisms to account for the execution of controlled movement [Schmidt and Russell, 1972]," or that "... feedback from a particular preprogrammed movement does not play a role in the control of that movement [Schmidt, 1972]," the term "feedback" is used in a rather limited manner, its sole frame of reference being attributed to signals generated by the response. Proponents of the internal feedback hypothesis, however, view information generated within the central nervous system as no less significant than response feedback. It would seem that in the intricate sequence of actions and reactions making up a motor response, the necessity of correcting errors well before the emergence of the final output should be recognized. Internal feedback thus warrants some consideration in future models of motor control.

B. Behavioral Research

1. Clinical Studies on Perceptual Deficits

As indicated earlier, H.L. Teuber has been one of the major advocates of corollary discharge theory, spending a considerable part of his scientific career in the investigation of perception following brain injury and surgery, especially of the frontal lobe of the cerebral cortex. Recently, Teuber (1972) has reviewed the findings on a number of tasks designed to reveal perceptual deficits in patients with frontal lesions. One of the common features in such tasks is the requirement that the patient maintain his orientation under abnormal postural conditions. For example, normal subjects make only slight constant errors in setting a luminous line vertical under dark conditions where the head and body are tilted some 30°. Patients with frontal lobe lesions, on the other hand, make much larger errors, suggesting that they are unable to take their own posture and movements into account (Teuber and Mishkin, 1954). In addition, frontal damage has been demonstrated to lead to stimulus-bound behaviors in which patients exhibit (a) an inability to voluntarily release their grasp, and (b) a failure to predict the path of visual objects with eye or hand (Teuber, 1966, 1972).

These, and a variety of similar findings, have led to the notion that the principal role of frontal structures is to permit the organism to monitor his own movements in an anticipatory manner. This would imply that not only can we "... assimilate feedback from the periphery after the execution of particular motor acts, but that we should be able, by a feedforward type of mechanism, to predict the anticipated consequences of our action [Teuber, 1972, p. 639]." The "feedforward" takes the form of a central, corollary discharge, which, according to Teuber (1972, 1974), is the mechanism by which the CNS defines whether a movement is voluntary (self-produced) or involuntary (passive).

While Teuber's data suggest a role for some such mechanism, how can we test the hypothesis behaviorally? One prediction is that active movements, having the benefits of corollary discharge, should be of primary importance for perceptual development and sensorimotor coordination (Teuber, 1972). A way to shed some light on this issue would be to investigate the critical conditions under which normal subjects can adapt to a rearranged environment. On the basis of Teuber's hypothesis, active movement should be critical in the adaptation process.

2. Active Movement and Perceptual Adaptation

One of the primary reasons for studying perceptual adaptation is to discover the mechanisms by which the CNS adjusts to the growth of the body. How is this related to the notion of corollary discharge and self-produced movement? Clearly, as the body grows, the sensory inputs must be modified in accordance with the increased distance between the eyes and ears. More important for the present discussion, however, is that efferent signals must also alter in order to take into account the increased size of the limbs and musculature. Since "efference" is a unique aspect of self-produced movement, it follows that perceptual adaptation and normal sensorimotor functioning may also be contingent on self-produced movement.

Typically, in these investigations subjects view their hands through a prism which displaces the visual image by perhaps 11°. Prior to and following the exposure period, a measure of the subject's ability to localize a target is made. A comparison of the localization responses indicates that compensatory shifts occur only when the subject moves his hand actively during the period of prism exposure. The subject whose hand is passively moved by the experimenter reveals no such adaptive behavior (Held and Hein, 1963; Held, 1965). These and other similar findings (Held and Freedman, 1963) have led to a model of the adaptive process (Held, 1961) in which the neural commands to the muscles are monitored by an internal storage system which also receives the sensory feedback concurrent on those commands (reafference). The coupling of the output with the feedback signals at a central level is thought to be the necessary condition for adaptation to occur. Since in passive movements the motor outflow source is absent, little or no adaptation will occur (Held and Freedman, 1963). As Teuber (1972) points out, in referring to the foregoing data: "under such conditions only active exposure adapts; we would say that only active exposure involves corollary discharge and these discharges are the vehicle of normal adaptation [p. 646]."

Before accepting the Held and Teuber hypothesis we might ask if any other explanation could fit the data generated without necessarily evoking the concept of corollary discharge. It could be argued, for example, that the facilitation of prism adaptation by active as opposed to passive movement may have more to do with the allocation of attention and input dominance, rather than any specific contribution of corollary discharge. It seems likely that active movement may induce the subject to process the proprioceptive and prismatically determined visual locations of the arm. Since vision is dominant (Rock and Harris, 1972; Rock, 1966; Rock and Victor, 1964), the subject will attend to vision and proprioception will be recalibrated, i.e., the hand will come to feel where it is seen (Harris, 1965). With passive movement however, where the experimenter moves the subject's arm, there is really no need to process either the seen or felt location of the hand. The absence of attention to a specific input will be reflected by an absence of adaptation in Held's paradigm.

That attention plays an important role in perceptual adaptation is revealed in a recent experiment by Kelso et al. (1975a). When the task performed during the exposure period focussed attention on the visual input, the adaptive shift was entirely proprioceptive, a typical finding (Harris, 1965; Hay et al., 1965). However, when the subject was instructed to attend to proprioceptive location and ignore visual input, the adaptive shift was entirely visual. This finding, and earlier ones by Canon (1970, 1971) on visual-auditory discrepancy, suggest that attentional factors may determine the locus of adaptation to displaced vision.

In conclusion, it might be postulated that the roles of corollary discharge and attention in adaptation are not mutually exclusive. It could be that the presence or absence of corollary discharge determines the amount of attention devoted to a particular movement. One way to test this notion would be to force the subject to attend to the passively moved arm. If the hypothetical corollary discharge is necessary as an attention-inducing agent no significant adaptation should occur. On the other hand, if attentional factors operate independently of corollary discharge, adaptive shifts should occur. A further crucial experiment with regard to localizing the corollary discharge mechanism in the frontal cortex (Teuber, 1960, 1964, 1966, 1972; Evarts, 1971a) would be to study perceptual adaptation in patients with lesions of this structure. Theoretically it would be predicted that such patients should not adapt since the "vehicle of adaptation" would either be deficient or absent. It seems surprising that this research strategy has not been adopted.

3. Voluntary Movements and the Central Monitoring of Efference

a. Eye Movements. The most concrete support for the central control of movement comes from the work on eye movements dating as far back as von Helmholtz (1867). The argument, which has been often reviewed (Teuber, 1966; Merton, 1964; Festinger and Canon, 1965; Festinger *et al.*, 1967; Gyr, 1972; Goodwin *et al.*, 1972), is that the perceptual system obtains knowledge of eye position and movement via monitoring the efferent commands to the extra-ocular muscles rather than via proprioceptive feedback from muscle receptors. Unlike the proprioceptive modality, however, virtually no data exist on the psychophysical qualities of motor outflow information. What more direct evidence is there to support the usefulness of information based on efference? Festinger and Canon (1965) have demonstrated that subjects can locate a target light on the basis of saccadic movements more accurately than on the basis of smooth pursuit movements. The inference here is that saccadic movements are brought about in response to efferent signals concerning the known target position. With pursuit movements, on the other hand, the subject follows the target without knowing its final location, and therefore the efferent signals are less precise.

The role of efferent information in smooth pursuit eye movements has been recently investigated by Festinger and Easton (1974) using the Fujii illusion which typically causes a misperception of the path of movement. By careful monitoring of eye movements they were able to compare retinal information with the perception of the movement path of a light. It was argued that a discrepancy between the two should reflect the informational content of the monitored efferent commands available to the perceptual system. Since the orientation of the physical path of the visual target was always correctly perceived, it was concluded that the efferent command contained necessary directional information. However, the extent of the perceived path was always considerably less than the physical movement extent, suggesting that speed of pursuit movements was not monitored accurately by the efferent system. In summary, the eye movement data indicate that the monitored efferent command contains all the necessary information when the movement mode is saccadic, i.e., preprogrammed for extent and direction (Festinger and Easton, 1974), but rather limited information in the pursuit mode. But what of voluntary limb movements? Can the same arguments and logic be applied?

b. Limb Movements. One of the major attributes of the eye system is that the eye moves under a fairly constant set of forces provided by only two sets of muscles (the rectus and oblique muscles). It has been argued that as a result of the predictability of the forces involved, the efferent outflow can provide the necessary information about eye position. Within the skeletal system, however, the forces are usually always modified from movement to movement rendering prediction difficult, if not impossible. An efference-based mechanism has therefore been rejected as an accurate means of movement control in favor of a closed-loop system stressing sensory feedback (e.g., Adams, 1971).

Very recently, however, Jones (1972, 1974a,b,c) revived Lashley's (1917, 1951) notion that voluntary limb movements are predominantly controlled by motor outflow. Relying primarily on the deafferentation data of Taub and Berman (1968) on monkeys and the foregoing arguments derived from eye movement research, Jones rejected a role for proprioceptive feedback in motor control. When the subject makes a voluntary movement "as rapidly as possible," it is posited that the resulting efferent discharge is centrally monitored and stored as an efference copy (von Holst, 1954), which is thought to be a motor memory storage system operating without the requirement of peripheral feedback. The support for Jones' central monitoring of efference (CME) model comes from the finding that subjects can duplicate voluntary movements more accurately than constrained or passive movements. Under the latter conditions, where the subject moves to an experimenter-defined stop, it is argued that the subjects are dependent on joint inflow since they lack the opportunity to make a preset movement. Thus, because proprioceptive feedback has "no access to central mechanisms [Jones, 1974a, p. 38] " memory loss occurs.

One problem with Jones' hypothesis is that it fails to accommodate the literature in short-term motor memory (STMM), indicating that terminal location information can be retained under constrained conditions (Laabs, 1973; Marteniuk, 1973; Keele and Ells, 1972). In addition, interpolated processing activity during a retention interval leads to an increase in recall error, suggesting that location cues do require central capacity. Jones' main argument for CME as opposed to proprioceptive location cues rests on the finding that subjects duplicate movement extents (i.e., distance) equally well from variable and constant starting positions (Jones, 1974a). Hence, as long as the efferent commands for movement extent are the same for criterion and recall movements no deficits in motor recall occur, regardless of initial starting position. But what happens when the subject is forced to generate a different efferent output at recall from that employed from the criterion movement?

One of our experiments (Stelmach et al., 1975c, experiment 1) examined this question by comparing the reproduction of either the end point or the distance of a voluntary (preselected) movement. It was argued that the former condition, by rendering distance unreliable, would require the subject to alter his efference for the recall movement. According to Jones' (1974a) hypothesis, this procedure should result in less accurate recall, while distance reproduction should be superior since the efferent output for criterion and recall movements remained the same. As Figure 1 shows, the results militated against the Jones' hypothesis,

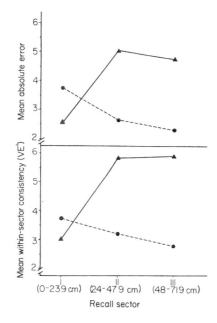

Figure 1 Mean absolute error and within-sector consistency (in cm) for preselected distance (▲) and location (●) conditions as a function of movement extent.

the location condition evidencing relatively less variability and absolute error after a 15-sec retention interval. This finding was congruent with studies in short-term motor memory and seemed to suggest that proprioceptive location cues were primary for accurate recall.

However, a subsequent experiment presented earlier (see Section II,A) indicated that proprioceptive information obtained at the end point of the movement was not the only factor involved. Providing the subject the opportunity to preselect a location prior to movement initiation also appears to be an important element in recall accuracy. It is feasible, therefore, that the combination of efferent and afferent information sources results in a stronger central representation relative to movement conditions where preselection is not available.

One way to examine the foregoing notion would be to introduce information reduction activity during the retention interval (Peterson and Peterson, 1959). If preselected location requires more central processing capacity, interpolated activity should differentially affect error compared to constrained and passive location conditions. Our data have failed to confirm this prediction, however, at least for rapid movements (Stelmach *et al.*, 1975c, experiment 3). While preselected location had significantly less absolute error than constrained and passive location, processing activity affected all conditions similarly, as revealed in Figure 2. This result is discrepant with Jones' (1974a) data where the

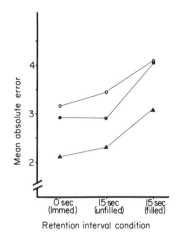

Retention interval condition

Figure 2 Mean absolute error (in cm) for preselected (▲), constrained (●), and passive (○) location conditions, as a function of retention interval condition.

preselected condition experienced greater error relative to constrained conditions when verbal processing was introduced. In addition, that constrained and passive location conditions were also affected by central processing activity is contrary to Jones' (1974a,b,c) argument that proprioceptive information fails to access central mechanisms, but is in agreement with the recent STMM literature (e.g., Laabs, 1973).

Viewed overall, our experiments contradict the CME hypothesis at least as conceptualized by Jones (1972, 1974a,b,c). Subjects *can* process proprioceptive information in constrained movements and they are not limited to the monitoring of an efference copy containing only movement extent information. Rather the data might suggest that preselection allows the subject to generate efferent impulses to a central representation of spatial location (MacNeilage, 1970; MacNeilage and MacNeilage, 1973; Russell, 1974, and Chapter 3 of this volume).

While the foregoing interpretation might at first seem plausible, our findings extend beyond the notion of a "central response organization unit to generate the motor commands which will result in movement to [a] location [Russell, 1974]." For example, Stelmach *et al.* (1975b) have shown that distance information can be encoded provided the subject is given the opportunity to preselect a desired movement extent. This finding is contrary to Marteniuk and Roy's (1972) suggestion that distance cues are "uncodable," but is in agreement with Jones (1974a) and a recent study by Diewert (1974). Furthermore, it cannot be argued that preselection is unique to rapid, "ballistic" movements which are preprogrammed and executed independent of peripheral control (e.g., Schmidt, 1972). One of our experiments has demonstrated that preselected movements are clearly superior in a slow positioning task. While constrained movements evidenced increased absolute and variable error over 15 sec, preselected movements remained stable (Stelmach *et al.*, 1975a).

Clearly, this phenomenon which we have called "preselection" has an overwhelming influence on movement reproduction, and would seem to be an important element in motor control. But what is the nature of preselection, and can it be accommodated by any of the control mechanisms discussed thus far in this chapter? Several hypotheses suggest themselves which appear to invite some speculation.

c. Preselection: Theoretical Implications and Possible Experiments. It seems likely that the availability of preselection allows the performer to internally organize or "plan" his response (Miller *et al.*, 1960) prior to movement initiation. In spite of providing the subject with what is thought to be the most salient form of information for coding movement, namely, afferent location cues (Laabs, 1973), an additional superiority of preselection is found. One way to examine the "plan" notion would be to determine if the act of preselection per se, is more attention-demanding than simply preparing to move to a constrained location. It might be predicted that the hypothesized response organization would require more attention and hence may cause an increase in probe reaction time (Ells, 1973) during the period in which the subject is instructed to select a movement.

An even more interesting question is whether preselection bears any relationship to corollary discharge. It could be postulated that the availability of preselection allows the performer to preset sensory systems in the manner alluded to by Teuber (1972). This would necessarily imply that preselection is related to self-produced movement as opposed to being simply a movement plan or strategy. The hypothesis could be tested by employing conditions which differ with regard to hypothesized outflow information (active versus passive) but are similar with regard to preselection. Thus, subjects in a preselected-active condition would actively move to a desired endpoint, while the preselected-passive condition would have the subject instruct the experimenter as to the desired end point of the passively moved limb. Differences between the conditions would imply that preselection may play a corollary discharge function. However a failure to obtain differences might suggest that preselection plays more of a cognitive role as opposed to being a unique aspect of voluntary, self-produced movement. Also, if one of the roles of preselection is to allow the subject to obtain prior knowledge of the movement, a failure to obtain differences might further bring into question the role of motor outflow. Since, according to Jones (1972), "for the perception of movement to be served by outflow, the subject would need to know the goal of his movement in advance [p. 95]." Knowing the goal and generating the motor output may in fact be independent functions in the initiation of a motor response.

Perhaps a final implication of our preselection data pertains to the role of sensory feedback. Since preselection occurs prior to movement, it is tempting to look upon it more in terms of a response or "output" code which may allow the organism to predict the outcome of the motor response independent of sensory factors. As MacNeilage and MacNeilage (1973) propose, "the *need* [italics theirs] for peripheral sensory feedback can be thought of as inversely proportional to the ability of the central nervous system to predictively determine without sensory information, every essential aspect of following acts [p. 424]." If preselection does allow us to "predictively determine" a motor response, sensory feedback may, as MacNeilage and MacNeilage suggest, play a relatively minor role. To investigate this hypothesis it would be necessary to examine voluntary movements in the absence of sensory feedback, the most important source of which is probably joint receptors (Skoglund, 1973; see Section II,A).

A less drastic method, however, might involve providing additional sources of input such as vision, which has been demonstrated to improve recall accuracy (Adams *et al.*, 1972), presumably by strengthening the memory trace (Adams and Goetz, 1973; Stelmach and Kelso, 1975). If the "code" of preselection is purely internal, operating prior to movement, additional visual information provided after the movement has begun should not aid reproduction. If reproduction improved, however, this would imply that the efferent information regarding the movement and the sensory feedback following the movement can interact. Such a finding would indicate that preselected movements are not merely coded in output terms. Rather the availability of preselection may allow the subject to encode afferent cues more effectively.

In summary, the foregoing experiments have examined the presetting of movement in order to determine if prior information about movements aids recall. As such they deviate from contemporary research approaches which have emphasized the role of sensory input in determining future motor acts. As Sperry (1969) has pointed out, however, any formulation regardless of its complexity in which sensory information is routed through central mechanisms into a motor response, becomes misleading. While the importance of peripheral information has not been excluded by the present experiments, they do however point to the potency of preselection in determining the accuracy of motor behavior. With the rejuvenation of interest into the neurophysiological mechanisms of movement control, it may be that, as Evarts (1971a) and others (Teuber, 1974; Sperry, 1969) have argued, the time has come to analyze behavior in terms of the organization of motor output as well as its relationship to sensory input.

IV. Concluding Comments

The major challenge facing researchers of human motor control lies in elucidating the manner in which central and peripheral processes interact in coordinating movements. It is misleading to assume that sensory feedback, important though it may be, is always necessary to elicit further motor output. Equally unrealistic is the notion that neural networks within the CNS generate stored movement patterns in total independence of peripheral feedback. Both peripheral and central approaches, if accepted in isolation of each other, leave too many questions unanswered.

Although drawing from some recent neurophysiological findings, the present approach has been primarily behavioral in its orientation. This, as was pointed out at the beginning, reflects the so-called switch in emphasis in motor skill research from a "product"- to a "process"-oriented approach wherein the underlying processes and mechanisms are of primary concern. The major problem, however, is that psychologists are still measuring product most of the time, rather than process. While the presence of certain processes may be inferred on occasion by measuring reproduction error, they cannot be explicated. Only by developing more analytical indices of performance can we expect to reveal underlying mechanisms. In this regard, the combination of psychological and neurophysiological methods is desirable. Progress has already been made with this approach, as evidenced in Evarts' (1973) work on learned movements in highly corticalized monkeys, and in Vallbo's (1971) development of a technique for recording from human muscle spindles. In both cases, the elicited motor behavior can be related to intervening neurophysiological phenomena, hopefully with the development of theory as the end result.

In advocating this approach, the intention is not to negate the individual contributions that the disciplines of psychology and neurophysiology can make to understanding human movement. As the present chapter suggests, however, the field of motor control, like the fields of sensory psychology and attention (Posner, 1974), can benefit from close ties between motor performance studies and neurophysiological explorations.

Acknowledgments

The preparation of this manuscript was supported in part by grants MH 22081-01 from the National Institute of Mental Health, NE-G-00-3-0099 from the National Institute of Education, and by the Graduate School of the University of Wisconsin awarded to George E. Stelmach. The opinions expressed herein do not necessarily reflect the position or policies of any of the above granting agencies.

References

Adams, J.A. (1971). *J. Mot. Behav.* 3, 111–150.
Adams, J.A. (1972). *Can. Psycho-Mot. Learn. Sport Psychol. Meet., 4th, 1972.*
Adams, J.A., and Goetz, E.T. (1973). *J. Mot. Behav.* 5, 217–224.

Adams, J.A., Goetz, E.T., and Marshall, P.H. (1972). *J. Exp. Psychol.* **92**, 291–297.

Allen, G.I., and Tsukahara, N. (1974). *Physiol. Rev.* **54**, 957–1006.

Andersson, S.A., Landgren, S., and Wolsk, D. (1966). *J. Physiol. (London)* **183**, 576–591.

Bahrick, H.P. (1957). *Psychol. Rev.* **64**, 324–328.

Bell, C. (1826). *Phil. Trans. Roy. Soc. London* **116**, 163–173.

Bossom, J. (1974). *Brain Res.* **21**, 285–296.

Bossom, J., and Ommaya, A.K. (1968). *Brain* **91**, 161–172.

Boyd, I.A. (1954). *J. Physiol. (London)* **74**, 469–488.

Brindley, G.S., and Merton, P.A. (1960). *J. Physiol. (London)* **153**, 127–130.

Browne, K., Lee, J., and Ring, P.A. (1954). *J. Physiol. (London)* **126**, 448–458.

Canon, L.K. (1970). *J. Exp. Psychol.* **84**, 141–147.

Canon, L.K. (1971). *J. Exp. Psychol.* **88**, 403–408.

Chase, R.A. (1965). *J. Nerv. Ment. Dis.* **140**, 239–251.

Christina, R.W., and Price, H.L. (1973). *Can. Congr. Multidisc. Study Sport Phys. Act., 1st, 1973.*

Coggeshall, R.E., Coulter, J.D., and Willis, W.D. (1973). *Abstr. Proc. Neurosci. Soc.* p. 387.

Cushman, P.G. (1958). *In* "Control Engineers' Handbook," pp. 2-3 to 2-56. McGraw-Hill, New York.

De Jong, R.N. (1951). "The Neurologic Examination." Harper (Hoeber), New York.

DeLong, M. (1971). *Neurosci. Res. Program, Bull.* **9**, 10–30.

Diewert, G.L. (1974). *Can. Psycho-Mot. Learn. Sport Psychol. Meet., 6th, 1974.*

Docherty, D. (1973). Ph.D. Thesis, University of Oregon, Eugene.

Doty, R.W. (1968). *In* "Handbook of Physiology" (Amer. Physiol. Soc., J. Field, ed.), Sect. 6, Vol. IV, pp. 1861–1902. Williams & Wilkins, Baltimore, Maryland.

Duchenne, G.B. (1883). "Selections from the Clinical Works of Dr. Duchenne." New Sydenham Society, London.

Eccles, J.C. (1973). "The Understanding of the Brain." McGraw-Hill, New York.

Eccles, J.C., Ito, M., and Szentagóthai, J. (1967). "The Cerebellum as a Neuronal Machine." Springer-Verlag, Berlin and New York.

Eklund, G., and Skoglund, S. (1960). *Acta Physiol. Scand.* **49**, 184–191.

Ells, J.G. (1973). *J. Exp. Psychol.* **99**, 10–21.

Evarts, E.V. (1971a). *Neurosci. Res. Program, Bull.* **9**, 86–112.

Evarts, E.V. (1971b). *Int. J. Neurol.* **8**, 321–326.

Evarts, E.V. (1972a). *Brain Res.* **40**, 25–31.

Evarts, E.V. (1972b). *In* "Corticothalamic Projections and Sensorimotor Activities" (T. Frigyesi, E. Rinuik, and M.D. Yahr, eds.), pp. 449–458. Raven Press, New York.

Evarts, E.V. (1973). *Science* **179**, 501–503.

Evarts, E.V., and Tanji, J. (1974). *Brain Res.* **71**, 479–494.

Evarts, E.V., and Thach, W.T. (1969). *Annu. Rev. Physiol.* **31**, 451–497.

Evarts, E.V., Bizzi, E., Burke, R.E., DeLong, M., and Thach, W.T. (1971). *Neurosci. Res. Program, Bull.* **9**, 1–170.

Festinger, L., and Canon, L.K. (1965). *Psychol. Rev.* **72**, 373–384.

Festinger, L., and Easton, A.M. (1974). *Psychol. Rev.* **81**, 44–58.

Festinger, L., Ono, H., Burnham, C.A., and Bamber, D. (1967). *J. Exp. Psychol.* **74**, Suppl., 1–36.

Gelfan, S., and Carter, S. (1967). *Exp. Neurol.* **18**, 469–473.

Gentile, A.M. (1972). *Quest* **17**, 3–23.

Giaquinto, S., Pompeiano, O., and Swett, J.E. (1963). *Arch. Ital. Biol.* **101**, 133–148.

Gibbs, C.B. (1954). *Brit. J. Physiol.* **56**, 233–242.

Goodwin, G.H., McCloskey, D.I., and Matthews, P.B.C. (1972). *Brain* **95**, 705–748.

Granit, R. (1955). "Receptors and Sensory Perception." Yale Univ. Press, New Haven, Connecticut.

Granit, R. (1970). "The Basis of Motor Control." Academic Press, New York.

Granit, R. (1972). *Brain* 95, 649–660.

Granit, R. (1973). *In* "Motor Control" (A.A. Gydikov, N.T. Taukov, and D.S. Kosarov, eds.), pp. 1–13. Plenum, New York.

Granit, R., and Burke, R.E. (1973). *Brain Res.* 53, 1–28.

Gyr, J.W. (1972). *Psychol. Bull.* 77, 246–261.

Hagbarth, K.E., and Vallbo, A.B. (1968). *Exp. Neurol.* 22, 674–694.

Harris, C.S. (1965). *Psychol. Rev.* 72, 419–444.

Hay, J.C., Pick, H.L., and Ikeda, K. (1965). *Psychonom. Sci.* 2, 215–6.

Held, R. (1961). *J. Nerv. Ment. Dis.* 132, 26–32.

Held, R. (1965). *Sci. Amer.* 213, 84–94.

Held, R., and Freedman, S.J. (1963). *Science* 142, 455–462.

Held, R., and Hein, A. (1963). *J. Comp. Physiol. Psychol.* 56, 872–876.

Higgins, J.R., and Angel, R.W. (1970). *J. Exp. Psychol.* 84, 412–416.

Hoff, P.A. (1971). *Percept. & Psychophys.* 9, 118–120.

Hollingworth, H.L. (1909). *Arch. Psychol.* 2, 1–87.

Hopkins, B. (1972). *Percept. Mot. Skills* 34, 431–435.

Howard, I.P., and Templeton, W.B. (1966). "Human Spatial Orientation." Wiley, New York.

Ito, M. (1970). *Intern. J. Neurol.* 7, 162–176.

Ito, M. (1974). *In* "The Neurosciences Third Study Program" (F.O. Schmitt and F.G. Worden, eds.), pp. 293–303. MIT Press, Cambridge, Massachusetts.

Jones, B. (1972). *Percept. & Psychophys.* 12, 95–96.

Jones, B. (1974a). *J. Exp. Psychol.* 102, 37–43.

Jones, B. (1974b). *J. Mot. Behav.* 6, 33–45.

Jones, B. (1974c). *Develop. Med. Child Neurol.* 16, 620–628.

Keele, S.W. (1973). "Attention and Human Performance." Goodyear, Pacific Palisades, California.

Keele, S.W. (1974). *Mot. Learn. Symp., 125th Anniv., Univ. Wis., Madison, Wis.*

Keele, S.W., and Ells, J.C. (1972). *J. Mot. Behav.* 4, 127–134.

Kelso, J.A.S. (1973). M.S. Thesis, University of Wisconsin, Madison.

Kelso, J.A.S., Stelmach, G.E., and Wanamaker, W.M. (1974). *J. Mot. Behav.* 6, 179–190.

Kelso, J.A.S., Cook, E., Olson, M.E., and Epstein, W. (1975a). *J. Exp. Psychol.* 1, 237–245.

Kelso, J.A.S., Wallace, S.A., Stelmach, G.E., and Weitz, G.A. (1975b). *Quart. J. Exp. Psychol.* 27, 141–147.

Konishi, M. (1965). *Z. Tierpsychol.* 22, 770–783.

Kornhuber, H.H. (1974). *In* "The Neurosciences: Third Study Program" (F.O. Schmitt and F.G. Worden, eds.), pp. 267–280. MIT Press, Cambridge, Massachusetts.

Laabs, G.E. (1973). *J. Exp. Psychol.* 100, 168–177.

Lashley, K.S. (1917). *Amer. J. Phys.* 43, 169–194.

Lashley, K.S. (1951). *In* "Cerebral Mechanisms in Behavior" (L.A. Jeffress, ed.), pp. 112–136. Wiley, New York.

Lashley, K.S., and Ball, J. (1929). *J. Comp. Psychol.* 9, 71–106.

Lashley, K.S., and McCarthy, D.A. (1926). *J. Comp. Psychol.* 6, 423–434.

Lassek, A.M. (1953). *J. Neuropathol. Exp. Neurol.* 12, 83–87.

Laszlo, J.I. (1966). *Quart. J. Exp. Psychol.* 18, 1–8.

Laszlo, J.I. (1967a). *Quart. J. Exp. Psychol.* 19, 344–349.

Laszlo, J.I. (1967b). *Physiol. & Behav.* 2, 359–365.

Laszlo, J.I., and Bairstow, P.J. (1971). *J. Mot. Behav.* 3, 241–252.

Laszlo, J.I., Shamoon, J.S., and Sanson-Fisher, R.W. (1969). *J. Mot. Behav.* **1**, 195–209.

Levine, D., and Ommaya, A.K. (1974). *Arch. Neurol. (Chicago)* (in press).

Llinas, R. (1974). *Physiologist* **17**, 19–46.

McCloskey, D.I. (1973). *Brain Res.* **63**, 119–131.

MacKay, D.M. (1966). *In* "Brain and Conscious Experience" (J.C. Eccles, ed.), pp. 422–445. Springer-Verlag, Berlin and New York.

MacNeilage, P.F. (1970). *Psychol. Rev.* **77**, 182–196.

MacNeilage, P.F., and MacNeilage, L.A. (1973). *In* "The Psychophysiology of Thinking" (F.J. McGuigan and R.A. Schoonover, eds.), pp. 417–448. Academic Press, New York.

Marler, P. (1970). *J. Comp. Physiol. Psychol., Monogr.* **71**, 1–25.

Marr, D. (1969). *J. Physiol. (London)* **202**, 437–470.

Marsden, C.D., Merton, P.A., and Morton, H.B. (1972). *Nature (London)* **238**, 140–143.

Marsden, C.D., Merton, P.A., and Morton, H.B. (1973). *Lancet* **1**, 759–761.

Marteniuk, R.G. (1973). *J. Mot. Behav.* **5**, 249–259.

Marteniuk, R.G., and Roy, E.A. (1972). *Acta Psychol.* **36**, 471–479.

Marteniuk, R.G., and Ryan, M.L. (1972). *J. Mot. Behav.* **4**, 135–142.

Marteniuk, R.G., Shields, K.W., and Campbell, S.C. (1972). *Percept. Mot. Skills* **35**, 51–58.

Massion, J. (1973). *J. Physiol. (Paris)* **67**, 117A–170A.

Matthews, P.B.C. (1972). "Mammalian Muscle Receptors and Their Central Actions." Arnold, London.

Matthews, P.B.C. (1974). *Brain Res.* **71**, 535–568.

Matthews, P.B.C., and Simonds, A. (1974). *J. Physiol. (London)* **239**, 27P–28P.

Mayr, O. (1970). *Sci. Amer.* **223**, 110–118.

Merton, P.A. (1953). *In* "The Spinal Cord" (J.L. Malcolm and J.A.B. Gray, eds.), pp. 247–255. Churchill, London.

Merton, P.A. (1961). *J. Physiol. (London)* **156**, 555–577.

Merton, P.A. (1964). *Symp. Soc. Exp. Biol.* **18**, 387–400.

Merton, P.A. (1970). *In* "Breathing: Hearing-Breuer Centenary Symposium" (R. Porter, ed.), pp. 207–217. Churchill, London.

Merton, P.A. (1974). *Brain Res.* **71**, 475–478.

Miller, G.A., Galanter, E., Pribram, K.H. (1960). "Plans and the Structure of Behavior." Holt, New York.

Mott, F.W., and Sherrington, C.S. (1895). *Proc. Roy. Soc.* **57**, 481–488.

Mountcastle, V.B., and Powell, T.S. (1959). *Bull. Johns Hopkins Hosp.* **105**, 173–200.

Mountcastle, V.B., Covian, M.R., and Harrison, C.R. (1952). *Res. Publ., Ass. Res. Nerv. Ment. Dis.* **30**, 339–370.

Oscarsson, O. (1965). *Physiol. Rev.* **45**, 495–522.

Oscarsson, O. (1967). *In* "Neurophysiological Basis of Normal and Abnormal Activities" (M.D. Yahr and D.P. Purpura, eds.), pp. 93–117. Raven Press, New York.

Oscarsson, O. (1972). *Brain Res.* **40**, 99–102.

Paillard, J., and Brouchon, M. (1968). *In* "The Neuropsychology of Spatially Oriented Behavior" (S.J. Freedman, ed.), pp. 37–55. Dorsey, Homewood, Illinois.

Paillard, J., and Brouchon, M. (1974). *Brain Res.* **71**, 273–284.

Peterson, L.R., and Peterson, M.J. (1959). *J. Exp. Psychol.* **58**, 193–198.

Pew, R.W. (1974). *In* "Human Information Processing: Tutorials in Performance and Cognition" (B.H. Kantowitz, ed.), Erlbaum, New York.

Phillips, C.G. (1969). *Proc. Roy. Soc., Ser. B* **173**, 141–174.

Phillips, C.G. (1971). *Neurosci. Res. Program, Bull.* **9**, 135–139.

Posner, M.I. (1974). *In* "The Handbook of Psychobiology" (M.S. Gazzaniga and C. Blakemore, eds.), pp. 441–480. Academic Press, New York.

Pribram, K.H. (1971). *"Languages of the Brain." Prentice-Hall, Englewood Cliffs, New* Jersey.

Provins, K.A. (1958). *J. Physiol. (London)* **143**, 55–67.

Rock, I. (1966). "The Nature of Perceptual Adaptation." Basic Books, New York.

Rock, I., and Harris, C.S. (1972). *In* "Perception: Mechanisms and Models" (R. Held and W. Richards, eds.), pp. 269–277. Freeman, San Francisco, California.

Rock, I., and Victor, J. (1964). *Science* **143**, 594–596.

Ronco, P.G. (1963). *J. Psychol.* **55**, 227–238.

Rose, J.E., and Mountcastle, V.B. (1959). *In* "Handbook of Physiology" (Amer. Physiol. Soc., J. Field, ed.), Sect. 1, Vol. I, pp. 387–429. Williams & Wilkins, Baltimore, Maryland.

Rushworth, G. (1960). *J. Neurol., Neurosurg. Psychiat.* [N.S.] **23**, 99–118.

Russell, D.G. (1974). *N. Amer. Soc. Psychol. Sport Phys. Act.. 1974.*

Schmidt, R.A. (1969). *J. Exp. Psychol.* **79**, 43–47.

Schmidt, R.A. (1972). *Psychonom. Sci.* **27**, 83–85.

Schmidt, R.A. (1975). *Psychol. Rev.* **82**, 225–260.

Schmidt, R.A., and Gordon, G.B. (1974). *Can. Psycho-Mot. Learn. Sport Psychol. Meet., 6th, 1974.*

Schmidt, R.A., and McCabe, J.F. (1972). *Can. Psycho-Mot. Learn. Sport Psychol. Meet., 4th, 1972.*

Schmidt, R.A., and Russell, D.G. (1972). *J. Exp. Psychol.* **96**, 315–320.

Schmitt, F.O., and Worden, F.G., eds. (1974). "The Neurosciences: Third Study Program." MIT Press, Cambridge, Massachusetts.

Sears, T.A. (1974). *Brain Res.* **71**, 465–473.

Shambes, G.M. (1969). *Amer. J. Phys. Med.* **48**, 225–236.

Sherrington, C.S. (1906). "The Integrative Action of the Nervous System." Yale Univ. Press, New Haven, Connecticut.

Skoglund, S. (1956). *Acta Physiol. Scand.* **36**, Suppl. 124.

Skoglund, S. (1973). *In* "Handbook of Sensory Physiology, Somatosensory System" (A. Iggo, ed.), Vol. II, pp. 111–136. Springer-Verlag, Berlin and New York.

Smith, J.L. (1969). *In* "New Perspectives of Man in Action" (R.C. Brown and B.J. Cratty, eds.), pp. 31–48. Prentice-Hall, Englewood Cliffs, New Jersey.

Smith, J.L., Roberts, E.M., and Atkins, E. (1972). *Amer. J. Phys. Med.* **51**, 225–239.

Sperry, R.W. (1950). *J. Comp. Physiol. Psychol.* **43**, 482–489.

Sperry, R.W. (1969). *Psychol. Rev.* **76**, 532–536.

Stein, R.B. (1974). *Physiol. Rev.* **54**, 215–243.

Stelmach, G.E., and Kelso, J.A.S. (1975). *Memory & Cognition.* **3**, 58–62.

Stelmach, G.E., Kelso, J.A.S., and McCullagh, P.D. (1975a). *Memory & Cognition* (in press).

Stelmach, G.E., Kelso, J.A.S., and Wallace, S.A. (1975b). *N. Amer. Soc. Psychol. Sport Phys. Act. 1975.*

Stelmach, G.E., Kelso, J.A.S., and Wallace, S.A. (1975c). *J. Exp. Psychol.* **1**, 745–755.

Stevens, S.S. (1957). *Psychol. Rev.* **64**, 153–182.

Swett, J.E., and Bourassa, C.M. (1967). *J. Neurophysiol.* **30**, 530–545.

Swett, J.E., Bourassa, C.M., and Inoue, S. (1964). *Science* **145**, 1071–1073.

Taub, E., and Berman, A.J. (1968). *In* "The Neuropsychology of Spatially Oriented Behavior" (S.J. Freedman, ed.), pp. 173–192. Dorsey, Homewood, Illinois.

Taub, E., Perrella, P., and Barro, G. (1973). *Science* **181**, 959–960.

Teuber, H.-L. (1960). *In* "Handbook of Physiology" (Amer. Physiol. Soc., J. Field, ed.), Sect. 1, Vol. III, pp. 1595–1668. Williams & Wilkins, Baltimore, Maryland.

Teuber, H.-L. (1964). *In* "The Frontal Granular Cortex and Behavior" (J.M. Warren and K. Akert, eds.), pp. 410–444. McGraw-Hill, New York.

Teuber, H.-L. (1966). *In* "Brain and Conscious Experience" (J.C. Eccles, ed.), pp. 182–216. Springer-Verlag, Berlin and New York.

Teuber, H.-L. (1972). *Acta Neurobiol. Exp.* **32**, 615–656.

Teuber, H.-L. (1974). *Brain Res.* **71**, 533–568.

Teuber, H.-L., and Mishkin, M. (1954). *J. Psychol.* **38**, 161–175.

Thach, W.T. (1970a). *J. Neurophysiol.* **33**, 527–536.

Thach, W.T. (1970b). *J. Neurophysiol.* **33**, 537–547.

Thach, W.T. (1972). *Brain Res.* **40**, 89–97.

Twitchell, T.E. (1954). *J. Neurophysiol.* **17**, 239–252.

Vallbo, Å.B. (1971). *J. Physiol. (London)* **218**, 405–431.

Vallbo, Å.B. (1973). *In* "Motor Control" (A.A. Gydikov, N.T. Taukov, and D.S. Kosarov, eds.), Plenum, New York.

Vierck, C.J. (1971). *Neurosci. Soc. Meet. 1972.*

von Helmholtz, H. (1867). "Handbuch der physiologischen Optik." Voss, Leipzig.

von Holst, E. (1954). *Brit. J. Anim. Behav.* **2**, 89–94.

Welford, A.T. (1972). *Res. Quart.* **43**, 295–311.

Whiting, H.T.A. (1972). *Res. Quart.* **43**, 266–294.

Williams, H.G. (1969). *In* "New Perspectives of Man in Action" (R.C. Brown and B.J. Cratty, eds.), pp. 50–76. Prentice-Hall, Englewood Cliffs, New Jersey.

Williams, I.D. (1973). *Can. Congr. Multidisc. Study Sport Phys. Act., 1st, 1973.*

The Schema as a Solution
to Some Persistent Problems
in Motor Learning Theory

Richard A. Schmidt

I. Introduction

Over the past decades of research in motor behavior, there has been an increasing trend, as described by Pew (1974), away from a "task-oriented approach" toward a "process-oriented approach" to various problems in motor performance and learning. Earlier work focused primarily on the effect of various experimental variables on the performance of rather "global" motor responses (e.g., the effects of massed practice on the learning and performance of the pursuit rotor task), whereas recently there seems to be a shift in emphasis toward understanding the kinds of changes that occur in humans as they

41

perform and learn. This recent concern has led to the creation of various models and theories that attempt to explain performance data through the postulation of various hypothetical mechanisms or processes. The work of Adams (1971), Anokhin (1969), Bernstein (translated in 1967), Konorski (1967), Laszlo and Bairstow (1971), Pew (1974), and Sokolov (1969) are representative of this kind of thinking about motor skills. This trend has been important because it has stimulated a great deal of research and thinking about motor behavior that was not present in earlier traditions, and the area has become very interesting because of the competition among the various explanations of motor performance. This paper is concerned with the various theoretical approaches to the learning of motor skills. Some of the persistent problems for theory are discussed, and the Schmidt (1975a) schema theory is summarized, showing how some of these problems can be handled with this approach. Finally, some pressing concerns for future research and theorizing are presented.

II. Limitations of Existing Theories

A. The Storage Problem

In open-loop theories (or models) of learning and performance, movement control is assumed to be regulated by a central program that determines all of the relevant spatial and temporal details of a motor act such as a baseball swing (e.g., Henry and Rogers, 1960; Lashley, 1917). While open-loop theorists do not explicitly say so, there is the implication that for every response a subject makes, there is a separate motor program that controls it. The number of such programs for motor responding must be very large indeed when we consider the number of speeds that the person can move, the number of starting positions and environmental states that can exist prior to the response, and the number of spatial patterns that the response can take. The number of such programs has been estimated for speech production by MacNeilage and MacNeilage (1973); considering only English and the possible accents and inflections, there are approximately 100,000 different phonemes (sounds), each presumably requiring a separate program for its production. This presents a difficult theoretical problem in explaining how the CNS can store this many programs. While it is true that the neurological networks are extremely complex, and it is also true that there is no good evidence that this many programs cannot be stored, the storage problem has led many motor behaviorists away from the one-to-one motor program idea because it represents a rather unparsimonious approach to understanding human responding.

Postulating closed-loop systems, with the roles of feedback, error detection, and error correction strongly emphasized, does not solve the problem. If it is true (as Adams says in this volume; see Chapter 4) that movements are controlled via feedback and the reduction of error, there must be a reference of correctness against which each of the movements must be compared. Again considering the number of possible movements, this implies that there must be as many references of correctness with which response-produced feedback is compared as there are movements, leading again to the storage problem.

B. The Novelty Problem

This problem is related to the storage problem discussed above, but the concern here is production of novel movements. During a game, the basketball player performs a shot from the floor that has a combination of starting body position, goal distance, and environmental situation (position of other players, etc.) that, strictly speaking, he has never experienced previously, and thus the movement can be considered "novel." Bartlett recognized the novelty problem (although he did not call it that) when he discussed the movements involved in tennis:

> When I make the stroke I do not, as a matter of fact, produce something absolutely new, and I never merely repeat something old [Bartlett, 1932, p. 202].

Thus, although a given tennis stroke might appear to be identical to other strokes made previously, it is always somewhat different because of the particular situation under which it is to be performed. At the same time, it is not totally novel, being strongly related to other, similar movements made previously. There is little evidence concerning such novel movements, and some critics would argue that learning a tennis stroke would involve the learning of a limited number of motor programs (open-loop theory) or a limited number of references of correctness (closed-loop theory) with the player choosing the proper program or reference depending upon the particular circumstances; thus the resulting movement would not be novel at all. However, investigations using cinematography for analysis of movement (e.g., Higgins and Spaeth, 1972) have shown that movements performed under apparently identical environmental conditions result in slightly different movement patterns, and that two apparently identical movements are not exactly alike in the pattern of output.

The theoretical problem that the novelty problem raises is that if performers can produce movements that have never been exactly performed previously, where do the references of correctness or motor programs come from? One cannot argue that they come from previous practice of the movement, because that particular movement has not been practiced before, and neither can one profitably argue that they are genetically determined. This presents a difficult problem that has not been considered in the development of theories of motor control.

C. The Detection of Errors

A third persistent problem that has faced theorists in motor control is how the individual can come to recognize his own errors and to produce corrections in subsequent responses. The most popular approach has been the adoption of closed-loop theory, in which response-produced feedback is compared against a reference of correctness to generate an error, and the error is the stimulus for subsequent corrections, a solution adopted by Adams (1971), Pew (1974), and Sokolov (1969). With the exception of Adams' (1971) position, however, in each of these theories the commands for action are generated first, and only then is the reference against which feedback is to be compared generated. The important point is that the reference of correctness is generated as a result of choosing the movement commands, and represents the expected feedback consequences of producing that movement. Thus, the only error that the performer can detect is that he failed to execute the program effectively, perhaps because there was "noise" in the system or because there were unpredicted variations in the state of the environment (e.g., wind on the tennis racket) that prevented the movement from being carried out as planned. While it is possible to imagine the subject making an error caused by "noise" in the motor system, there are no data that indicate to what extent these errors occur in skills, or even if they occur at all. Even if they do occur, we have no evidence that subjects can learn to recognize these errors.

More important, however, is the fact that these theories cannot explain how the subject detects and corrects a second, and more critical, type of error: an error in which the environmental goal is not met. Even if the movement actually chosen were perfectly executed, the movement could be grossly incorrect because the intended movement did not match the environmental demands. In other words, the subject can choose the wrong movement and execute it correctly (receiving no error information according to the theories mentioned above), and can still produce an error because the movement did not meet the environmental demands. The detection of the extent to which the environmental goal of the movement is met, in contrast to the detection of error in execution, is well supported by the evidence, as Schmidt and White (1972) and Schmidt and Wrisberg (1973) have shown that subjects are able to accurately estimate their performance scores after a movement has been completed.

Adams (1971) recognized this difficulty with the earlier positions, and his theory has the reference of correctness separate from the generation of the movement, so that the feedback from the movement can be compared against the feedback that "should" arise if the movement is, in fact, achieving the environmental goal. Since Adams has the reference of correctness tied to the environmental goal of the movement (e.g., the criterion location of the lever in positioning) rather than to the choice of the commands to produce the movement, the theory provides a means whereby the subject can detect the exte. which the environmental goal was achieved. The resulting error information can be used during a positioning movement to produce subsequent corrections so that the limb is guided to the correct location via the reduction or error. This feature of the Adams theory enables it to account for a great deal of learning data that could not be handled by the earlier theories, and is therefore a very strong aspect of its theoretical position.

III. A Possible Solution: The Schema Theory

The Schmidt (1974, 1975a) schema theory evolved from an attempt to take the strong parts of various theoretical positions, adding modifications and extensions so that the new theory would be able to deal with some of the problems raised in the previous sections, particularly the storage and novelty problems. A strong lead was provided by Adams' (1971) theory which has had a large influence on motor behavior because (1) the theory deals with the learning of motor skills, while most other theories deal with performance, (2) the theory is tied strongly to empirical data, and (3) Adams suggests experimental paradigms that enable the theory to be tested in the laboratory. The result of these features has been a great deal of research activity testing Adams' theory in the short time since its publication. But a number of problems appeared for the theory as a result of the research and thinking that it generated. These difficulties are discussed in detail in Schmidt (1975a) and are only summarized briefly here.

First, Adams' theory cannot deal with either the novelty problem or the storage problem because it assumes that for every movement there is a reference of correctness against which response-produced feedback is compared during the response. Second, there are logical difficulties associated with the prediction that, in slow positioning tasks, the subject should acquire a strong capacity to recognize his errors after the movement, and should be able to substitute this subjective information for knowledge of results (KR); this does not logically follow from the theory, nor are there data that support this contention. And third, Williams and Rodney (1975, unpublished) have presented evidence contrary to the prediction that in order to develop the reference of correctness (Adams' perceptual trace) the subject must have moved to the goal position previously (see Section IV,A,2 for a discussion of this study).

The schema theory postulates two separate states of memory, one for recall and one for recognition, as Adams' theory had done. The specific roles of recall and recognition memory depend slightly upon the type of task, but basically recall memory is the state responsible for the generation of impulses to the musculature that carry out movement (or movement corrections), while recognition memory is the state responsible for evaluation of response-produced feedback that makes possible the generation of error information about the movement.

It is also assumed that there are "generalized" motor programs formed in the central nervous system that contain stored muscle commands with all of the details necessary to carry out a movement. The program requires response specifications that determine how the program is to be carried out (e.g., rapidly, slowly, etc.). Given the response specifications, the program can be run off, with all of the details of the movement determined in advance.

The role of the program varies depending upon the duration of the movement. If the movement is rapid (i.e., with a movement time of less than 200 msec), the movement is carried out under the complete control of recall memory, in that the program determines all of the details of the movement in advance, and any event in the environment that signals that the present movement should be changed must await one reaction time before a new program can begin to become effective. Thus, in rapid movements, where the movement time is frequently less than one reaction time, the subject carries out the already programmed movement even though the environment might later indicate that this movement will be incorrect. Recognition memory operates after the movement is completed, providing expected sensory consequences against which the response-produced feedback stimuli are compared, with any resulting discrepancies indicating that an error has occurred.

With slower movements, such as linear positioning tasks, the movement is carried out using both recall and recognition. Here, the subject makes short programmed moves along the track, and after each one he compares the response-produced feedback against the expected sensory consequences. If the two do not match, a corrective movement is provided, the comparison is again made, and so on until the difference between the expected sensory consequences and the response-produced feedback is zero. Thus, the role of recall memory is to produce small, adjustive movement only, and the primary determinant of accuracy in the task is the comparison of expected and actual feedback. Hence, slow movements are dependent on recognition memory, even though the subject might be making adjustive responses with recall memory.

The theory also indicates how the response specifications and expected sensory consequences are generated. When the subject makes a movement, he stores a number of separate pieces of information. First, he stores the response specifications used for that movement. Second, he stores the initial conditions that existed when the movement was begun, including the individual's location in space, the relative positions of his limbs, and the state of the environment. Third, the subject stores the actual outcome of the movement, usually determined by the information presented by the experimenter in the form of KR, but sometimes resulting from the subject's own evaluation of the outcome of his movements (e.g., he saw the ball hit the target). And finally, he stores the sensory consequences of the movement, that is, the exteroceptive and proprioceptive consequences of making the response. Given these four sources of information, the theory assumes the development of a recall schema and a recognition schema that form the basis of the two states of memory.

A. The Schema Defined

The recall schema is the relationship, built up over past experience, between the actual outcome and the response specifications. When the subject makes a movement, he pairs the response specifications and the actual outcome on that particular trial. After a number of such attempts, there begins to form a relationship between two variables, and this relationship (the recall schema) is updated on each successive trial. After a great deal of experience the schema becomes well established. When the subject attempts to produce a novel movement he enters the schema with the desired outcome and the initial conditions, and the schema rule produces the response specifications for that movement. When the response specifications have been determined, the movement can be carried out by running the motor program.

The recognition schema operates in an analogous way, but the variables of concern are initial conditions, sensory consequences, and actual outcomes (KR). On each trial, the sensory consequences and actual outcome are paired, and are used to develop the relationship between sensory consequences and actual outcome (which is the recognition schema).[1] During an actual movement, the subject can specify the desired outcome and, through the recognition schema, can predict the expected sensory consequences of the movement. Then, after a rapid movement, the actual sensory consequences are compared with the expected sensory consequences, with any discrepancy indicating that an error has occurred in the movement. In this way the subject can have information about the correctness of his movements without having to be given KR. In the absence of KR, the error signaled by the recognition schema can be substituted for actual outcome information, and can allow the further updating of the recall schema; thus, the subject can learn without KR if the recognition schema is sufficiently well developed. Also, it should be noted that after a slow movement, where accuracy is controlled by recognition memory, the subject cannot generate error information about the success of his movement since he has stopped at that position for which his error signal was equal to zero; hence, there can be no

---

[1] In both the recognition and recall schemas, initial conditions are a third variable in the schema rule. Thus, it would be better to say that the recall schema is the relationship among responses specifications, actual outcomes, and initial conditions, and that the recognition schema is the relationship among sensory consequences, actual outcomes, and initial conditions.

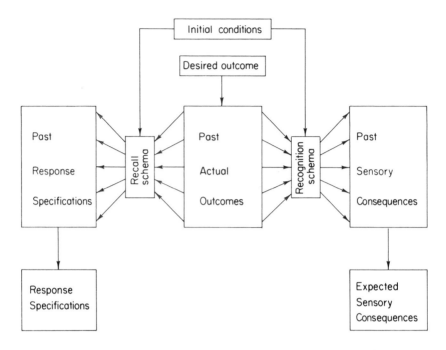

Figure 1 The recall and recognition schema in relation to various sources of information. (From Schmidt, 1975a.)

subjective reinforcement, and no learning without KR, in slow responses. The recall and recognition schemas are depicted in Figure 1; Figure 2 shows how the two schemas are thought to fit into the overall motor system, their interaction with feedback of various types, and the flow of information within a trial.

B. The Schema and Learning

It is important to define how the schemas are developed with practice. Since, for example, the recall schema is the relationship built up over trials between response specifications and actual outcomes (as modified by initial conditions), the strength of the schema is assumed to be a positive function of (a) the number of such pairs experienced (i.e., the number of prior trials) and (b) the variability of such prior experiences. Increased amount and variability in such experiences will lead to the development of an increasingly strong recall schema, so that when the subject is transferred to a novel situation governed by the schema, he will be able to determine more effectively the appropriate response specifications given the desired outcome and the initial conditions. In addition to improved performance on the first trials of the novel movement, the theory

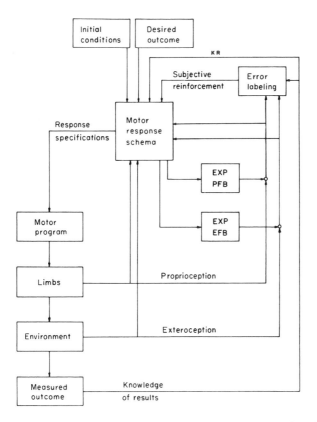

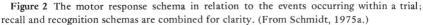

Figure 2 The motor response schema in relation to the events occurring within a trial; recall and recognition schemas are combined for clarity. (From Schmidt, 1975a.)

predicts increased rate of learning for the new task as a function of increased variability in previous movement experiences.

A similar argument holds for the recognition schema. Increased variability in practice leads to a stronger relationship between the actual outcome and the sensory consequences (as modified by the initial conditions). Then, when the recognition schema has been developed over practice, on a novel rapid movement the subject can generate the expected sensory consequences of that movement (even though he may never have performed it previously), and can compare the actual and expected sensory consequences to determine the extent of error on that trial; on a novel slow movement, the subject can move to the correct position through the comparison of response-produced feedback and the expected sensory consequences as generated by the recognition schema. Thus, increased variability in practice leads to increased sensitivity for estimating the outcome of the movement just made; if KR is not present in a fast movement, then the subject can inform himself about his errors via the recognition schema, and can make adjustments even without external error information.

C. The Schema and the Storage-Novelty Problems

The schema theory provides a solution to the storage problem for motor skills by postulating that the subject stores the relationship between actual outcomes, sensory consequences, and initial conditions for the recognition schema, and the relationship between actual outcomes, response specifications and initial conditions for the recall schema. These values that form the relationship are only stored briefly, however, and do not remain in memory except as they are needed to update the schema rules after the movement is completed. There is evidence from the pattern-recognition literature (e.g., Posner and Keele, 1970) that subjects store an abstraction of the set of patterns observed (the schema) as well as the individual patterns themselves, but the abstraction is retained more effectively over time than are the individual patterns, avoiding the theoretical problem of having all of the individual patterns being stored in permanent memory.

To produce a novel movement, the subject begins with the initial conditions and the desired outcome. Given these two sources of information, he "interpolates" between past outcomes (as modified by the initial conditions) to determine the response specifications that should be produced if the desired outcome is to be met. Thus, the subject can choose a completely novel set of response specifications that will result in a novel movement. Notice that there is no necessity for a specific motor program to be stored for each movement that the subject makes, and that the schema in conjunction with the generalized motor program can specify the response specifications for a large number of movements of this type.

A similar argument holds for recognition memory, but in this case the schema is the relationship between sensory consequences and actual outcomes, as modified by the initial conditions. When the subject makes a novel movement, having the desired outcome and initial conditions specified allows the schema to generate the expected sensory consequences of that movement, even though that movement may never have been made before. Then, if the movement is rapid (e.g., movement time less than 200 msec), the expected sensory consequences are compared with the actual sensory consequences to define an error, which can be substituted for KR to guide changes in the response on the next trial. If the movement is slow (e.g., a positioning response), then the difference between the actual and expected sensory consequences defines an error that can be responded to within the same movement, and the subject moves to that position he recognizes as correct (i.e., as having zero error). In either case, the recognition schema can satisfy the novelty and storage problems because (a) there is no necessity of storing the sensory consequences for every past movement, and (b) the subject can produce a novel slow movement by matching the actual sensory consequences with the expected consequences, or he can recognize the correctness of the novel fast movement through the difference between expected and actual sensory consequences after the movement.

D. The Schema and Error Detection

Error information in the schema theory is generated by a comparison between the expected sensory consequences (generated from the recognition schema) and the response-produced sensory information. Earlier theories use this type of comparison to generate an error, but the main distinction between these and the schema theory concerns how the expected sensory consequences are chosen. In the schema theory, the subject begins with the desired outcome (the environmental goal) for the movement. Then the response specifications and the expected sensory consequences are generated from separate schemas: recall and recognition, respectively. These states are separate because they are developed using different sources of information. Both the recall and recognition schemas use actual outcomes and initial conditions, but the recall schema is the relationship between these two variables and the response specifications, whereas the recognition schema is the relationship between these two variables and sensory consequences. Thus, specifying a desired outcome enables the generation of response specifications and expected sensory consequences semi-independently. The expected sensory consequences represent the best estimate of the nature of the response-produced feedback that would be produced if the goal is achieved, while the response specifications represent the best estimate of the response specifications that will have to be used in order that the goal be achieved.

IV. Some Key Concerns Facing the Schema Theory

While the schema theory can provide solutions to a number of the common problems facing earlier motor-learning theories, the notion has a few difficulties of its own. This section discusses some of the most important problems facing the schema theory, and presents some possible means whereby the problems can be solved. The most serious question surrounding the schema theory is the apparent lack of evidence supporting the existence of motor schemas, and it is to this issue that we turn next.

A. Evidence for the Motor Schema

The strength of the evidence for the schema notion is quite different for the two types of schemas (recognition and recall) presented in the theory. The evidence for the recognition schema is quite strong indeed, but the support for the recall schema is somewhat lacking.

1. Recall Schema Evidence

Speaking subjectively, it makes a great deal of sense to infer that something like a recall schema must exist if we are able to produce a movement of a given class that we have never produced before. This argument, together with the unattractiveness of the theories that imply the storage of one motor program or reference of correctness for each movement that the subject will ever produce, makes attracitve the argument for a system that conserves storage space and enables flexibility. Of course, this kind of reasoning does not provide sufficient justification or evidence for the schema notion, but there are a few experiments that suggest the existance of a recall schema.

One of the major predicitions of the recall schema ideas is that increased variability in practicing a number of variations of a movement class should result in increased transfer to a new, and as yet unpracticed, member of that same class. This idea has been tested several times (e.g., Crafts, 1927; Duncan, 1958), and the evidence is reasonably clear that this prediction from the schema theory has held in earlier work. For example, Duncan (1958) used a task in which there were 13 slots into which a lever could be positioned, and the subject's task was to move the lever to the appropriate slot when one of the 13 light stimuli came on. Duncan constructed the task so that 12 variations of it could be produced, and he varied the number of different tasks (either 1, 2, 5, or 10) that were presented in training trials, holding the absolute number of trials constant. The amount of transfer to two novel variations of the same task (not used in the training trials) was a positive function of both the amount and variability in training, providing evidence for the schema theory predictions.

While it might seem that this evidence could be interpreted as showing the development of a recall schema for the class of tasks in question, the task had substantial cognitive components, with the primary task for the subject being to learn which of the 13 responses went with the various stimuli; the actual movements of the lever seem quite trivial in contrast to these cognitive processes. The Duncan paper appears to show the existence of schemas for making decisions about light-slot pairings, which can be considered as a type of concept formation, but the important question here concerns the development of schemas that can provide the details necessary for the motor program to produce a novel set of motor commands, and the Duncan findings really do not provide such evidence. What was needed was an experiment using Duncan's basic design, but using a task in which it could not be argued that a cognitive concept only was being transferred, leaving the way clear for an interpretation in terms of a motor recall schema.

R.A. Schmidt and D. Shapiro (unpublished data, University of Southern California, 1974) conducted an experiment that used Duncan's (1958) method, but with a more "motor" task. The subject had to knock over four small barriers with the right hand in a predefined order, and the goal was to perform the task as rapidly as possible. The task could be varied by changing the locations of the barriers (but not their orders) to produce four different tasks, varying slightly in terms of the lengths of the movement segments and the angles between them. One group of subjects performed three of the tasks, 40 trials of each with KR after each trial, while a second group performed a single, randomly assigned task for 120 trials with KR. Thus the amount of practice on the task was constant, and variability in practice was the experimental variable. When subjects were transferred to the fourth task, the subjects with high variability in practice tended to perform the fourth task more rapidly, with differences increasing slightly as practice continued over the 40 task 4 trials; but these differences were quite small, and were not statistically reliable.

Data such as these do not, of course, disprove the existence of the schema, as the lack of significant advantage for the high-variability group might be explained by the fact that the task involved the dominant hand in ways that have been used in previous tasks throughout the subject's lifetime. Thus, the schemas for arm movements might have been well developed by the time the subjects entered the laboratory, rendering the added variability in laboratory activity relatively ineffective in generating further increases in schema strength. Also, it could be that the four variations were not sufficiently different, or were different in the "wrong" ways, for the development of added schema strength. These experiments should be attempted using more novel tasks, perhaps with younger children in whom such schemas would have more opportunity to be strengthened by laboratory activities.

Thus, while it is true that there is no strong experimental evidence that supports the existence of the recall schema notion, neither is there evidence against it. However, subjectively, we appear to be able to produce responses that we have not made before. If it is true that we can, then we need a notion like the schema to explain how these can be performed. The most important line of research that can be done in relation to the schema will therefore concern the verification of the existence of the recall schema.

2. Recognition Schema Evidence

In sharp contrast to the scanty evidence for the existence of the recall schema, there is considerable support for recognition schemas, although most of the evidence does not involve strictly motor tasks. The main point to be demonstrated in such experiments is that a subject can learn to recognize a stimulus that he has never experienced previously, and a number of experiments have shown that this can be done.

A good example of this type of demonstration is provided by Posner and Keele (1968, experiment III). They presented subjects a series of 9-dot patterns on a screen. There were three basic patterns termed "prototypes," and variations of the prototypes termed "distortions" were formed by randomly moving each of the 9 dots slightly. The experimenters presented 12 distortions (4 from each prototype) to subjects in a training session, and subjects learned with KR to classify the distortions into the correct category; the original prototypes were never presented in this session. In a transfer session, subjects received the 3 prototypes, 6 "old" distortions (2 from each prototype) from the training session, 12 "new" distortions (not previously shown), and 3 unrelated random patterns. Subjects were able to classify the prototypes (which they had not seen previously) nearly as accurately (14.9% errors) as the distortions that thay had seen previously (13.0% errors). The interpretation was that the presentation of the distortions in the training session enabled the subjects to develop a "concept" (or schema) concerning the 3 prototype dot patterns. Then, when the prototypes were presented, the subjects could recognize them even though they had not seen them previously. Similar findings have been shown by a number of other researchers as well (e.g., Attneave, 1957; Edmonds et al., 1966; Posner and Keele, 1968, 1970).

The important point for the present purposes is that these experiments have provided evidence, with visually presented materials, for a recognition schema that enables the subject to recognize and classify stimuli that he has not experienced previously. One way of thinking about the mechanisms behind the Posner-Keele (1968, 1970) findings is that the subject developed the schemas for the various prototypes during practice with the distortions. When a "new" stimulus is presented, the subject compares the stimuli against the schema for the prototype; if a match is received, the subject indicates that the stimuli are a member of the category. In the Schmidt (1975a) schema theory, a similar sort of process is thought to occur, and the Posner-Keele studies provide evidence for it. When the subject determines the desired outcome, the recognition schema generates the expected sensory consequences. When the movement is fired off, the response-produced sensory consequences are compared with the expected sensory consequences, and any mismatch signals that an error has occurred.

A study by Williams and Rodney (1975) provides additional evidence for the recognition schema. Subjects attempted to learn the criterion position for a linear-positioning task in two ways. One group moved 16 times to a stop that defined the position. A second group moved to stops at each of 16 randomly ordered positions to either side of the criterion, with subjects being told that the correct location lies in the center of this range. Then on transfer trials, all subjects attempted to move to the criterion position on 20 trials without the aid of either the stop or KR. Performances of the two groups (absolute errors) were nearly identical on the first transfer trial, but with additional trials the group with variability in practice maintained performance, while the group that moved to the stop regressed significantly. The interpretation in terms of the schema theory is that subjects could generate the expected sensory consequences of being in the correct location without ever having been at that position, and they could then match the actual and expected sensory feedback to position the lever at the correct location. While the Williams-Rodney data provide support for the recognition-schema notion, they also provide strong contradictory evidence for the Adams (1971) position. Adams' theory clearly predicts that the perceptual trace (the reference of correctness) develops as a function of having experienced the feedback stimuli resulting from being at the correct location, and that without having been at the correct location, the perceptual trace could not develop.

In contrast to the situation with the recall schema, there is rather strong evidence for the recognition schema idea. The evidence with visually presented stimuli provides encouragement that similar findings can be produced with stimuli presented in other modalities—such as proprioceptive or auditory—as well as for stimuli that represent errors in responding. In addition, the Williams-Rodney (1975) experiment provides evidence for the recognition schema for slow movements. Additional work needs to be done with other stimuli, and with more rapid motor tasks.

B. Some Problems with the Motor Program Concept

The evidence that Lashley's (1917) patient, who was accidentally deprived of sensation from his lower limbs by a gunshot wound, could position his limb rather "normally" stimulated the first suggestion that movement could be controlled centrally, without the need for peripheral feedback. Later various workers found that the time to process peripheral information was on the order of 150 msec (e.g., Posner and Keele, 1968; Slater-Hammel, 1960), raising questions about how the subject could possibly use peripheral feedback for the control of limb movements when the loop times were so long. A particular problem for closed-loop theorists was the fact that a subject can begin with the hand at rest, initiate a movement via an abrupt acceleration, and then decelerate the hand so that it comes to rest on a target 10 cm away, all with a movement time of 100 msec or less. The problem is where the "decelerate" instructions come from. If we wish to argue that the subject uses feedback to inform himself of his progress in the movement, such that when the movement reaches, for example, the halfway point the "decelerate" instructions are issued, we are faced with the problem that the movement is completed 50 msec or so before the "decelerate" instructions can even begin to become effective. Clearly, the instructions to stop the movement have to be planned prior to the beginning of the movement.

One solution to this problem was the postulation of the notion of the motor program, usually expressed as a set of prestructured movement commands that contain all of the details of the movement, including which muscles are to contract, for how long, and with what force. Keele's (1968) definition of the motor program as a set of prestructured muscle commands that allows movement to be carried out "uninfluenced by peripheral feedback [p. 387]" is the best accepted statement of the idea today. Various theorists have used the motor program as a largely "default" argument to provide a solution to the apparent fact that feedback loops are too slow to provide control in rapid movements (see, e.g., Pew, 1974), without insisting on direct evidence of the existence of the motor program.

There is evidence for a kind of motor programming with subhuman species. For example, Wilson (1961) has shown that locusts with deafferented wing systems can provide wing movements closely resembling the movements during flight in the intact insect, suggesting the existence of a motor program for wing movements. However, these programs are probably innate, and they might not indicate a great deal about the existence of learned motor programs such as would be necessary for a human to throw a ball. Because of the scant evidence for the program notion, there has been renewed controversy lately about its viability (e.g., Adams, this volume, Chapter 4), with other possibilities being proposed (Jones, 1971, 1974).

One major objection to the program notion as stated earlier is that evidence is accumulating that feedback is present in almost all movements, and that the loop time for the feedback to become effective may be far shorter then the 150–200 msec that is traditionally used. Consider, for example, the experiment by Dewhurst (1967), who had subjects hold a small weight in the hand, with the elbow flexed at $90°$, and monitored the EMG activity from the biceps. At a time unknown to the subject, the weight was suddenly either increased or decreased, resulting in a sudden displacement of the limb either downward or upward, respectively. Dewhurst showed that there was a change in the EMG pattern in approximately 30–50 msec, and that the limb began to reacquire its $90°$ position a short time thereafter. Similar findings have been produced with the chest musculature associated with breathing; when the resistance to the flow of air through a mouthpiece is suddenly increased, there is an increased EMG from the intercostal muscles within 30–80 msec (Sears and Newsom Davis, 1968). Findings such as these, not to mention the suggestion that loop times may be as rapid as 4–5 msec (Sussman, 1972) in the tongue, have been taken as evidence against the motor program notion that peripheral feedback is unnecessary in the control of movement.

The explanation for the corrections in the Dewhurst (1967) and Sears and Newsom Davis (1968) studies concerns the functioning of the muscle spindle system. There is good evidence (Granit, 1970) that the alpha efferent system (to the main body of the musculature) and the gamma efferent system (to the intrafusal muscle fibers of the muscle spindle) work in cooperation, and this concept is termed alpha-gamma coactivation. In the Dewhurst example, the argument is that the alpha and gamma systems are coactivated so they maintain the 90° position. The intrafusal fibers are "biased" so that if the position is altered by an external means, the spindles are changed in length, setting up a reflex change in the alpha activity (seen in the EMG patterns) for the biceps. These changes are quite rapid, and are known to have a loop time of approximately 30–50 msec, consistent with the findings in Dewhurst's (1967) experiment. In addition to such monosynaptic reflexes, there are higher-order reflexes as well (e.g., the "long-loop reflex") with somewhat longer times; these more "complex" reflexes, while being slower than the simple stretch reflex, are far faster than the usual 150-msec estimates of reaction time.

If alpha-gamma coactivation is used in the maintainance of posture, there is reason to believe that it is involved in the control of limb motion as well. For example, Smith (1969) showed that blockage of the gamma system with anesthetics impaired fine control in arm movements, and Frank (1975) has shown that the blockage of the stretch reflex via the cuff technique reduces fine control in finger movements even with vision presented.[2] In addition, Hubbard (1960) had subjects make oscillating elbow flexion movements at various speeds, and EMG records indicated that there were many alternating biceps and triceps contractions during a single movement (especially if the movements were very slow), with the time pattern of these contractions being consistent with the loop times for the spindle system. Evidence such as this suggests that the spindle, with alpha-gamma coactivation, may be strongly involved in the fine aspects of movement control.

The relevance of this evidence for the present argument about motor programs is that if central motor programs exist at all, it is clear that they must contain information not only to the main body of the musculature (i.e., the alpha efferent activity) but also the information to the intrafusal fibers of the muscle spindle (i.e., gamma efferent activity). In addition, reflex activity of the spindles appears to be present and active in most movements, and it therefore makes little sense to speak of the motor program as producing movements without involvement from peripheral feedback as Keele (1968) and others, including the writer (Schmidt, 1972; Schmidt and Russell, 1972), have done.

The problem for the motor program notion is not, therefore, whether or not feedback is active (because there is strong evidence that feedback is active), but rather it concerns what this feedback does in movement control. It is useful in this regard to define two kinds of errors whose corrections are based upon feedback. The first type of correction arises when something in the environment signals to the subject that the movement he has planned is not going to be

---

[2]These conclusions should be taken cautiously, however, because there was probably some decrement in alpha activity which could have reduced performance of the main musculature. However, since these tasks did not involve very much strength, an interpretation in terms of decrements in the gamma system seems reasonable.

correct. There are countless examples of this type of error, such as the ball changing course as the batter is swinging, seeing or feeling that one's limb is moving in the incorrect direction, and so on. There is very clear evidence that such stimuli, whether they result from the environment (ball-flight information) or whether they result from response-produced sources (seeing one's limb moving incorrectly), require one reaction time (about 150 msec at the least) for the subject to initiate a correction (e.g., Henry and Harrison, 1961; Keele and Posner, 1968; Slater-Hammel, 1960; see Schmidt, 1975b, for a discussion of this evidence). Thus, the movement that was planned carries itself out as if nothing had happened, and the movement is said to be programmed because the "originally intended" movement is carried out even though feedback might indicate that it is going to be incorrect. The generalization is that this type of error requires the subject to change the goal of the movement, such as swinging the bat in a different place, or moving the limb in a different direction.

The second type of error concerns situations in which sudden unexpected changed in the environment exert changes in the dynamics of the limb which, if uncorrected, will make the movement incorrect. For example, if in a tennis stroke an unexpected puff of wind slows the racket somewhat, the muscle-spindle system can exert a small correction to increase the output of the relevant musculature so that the "intended" swing is actually produced. Note that in this case the goal of the movement does not need to be changed (i.e., to swing at a given place and speed), but rather the spindle system needs to provide minor adjustments in the pattern of motor output for the given goal. These changes can be initiated very rapidly in sharp constrast to the 150-msec lags necessary to change the goal. Thus, this second type of error is in the execution of a movement, with the spindle system acting to ensure that the movement is carried out as "intended."

Those who argue, as Adams (Chapter 4 of this volume) has done, that feedback loop times can sometimes be very rapid—far more rapid than the 150-msec loop times usually accepted—are correct, but they fail to consider what kinds of corrections these sources of feedback are able to effect. If the implication is that the reflex activities of the spindle can effect a change in the goal of the movement within 30 msec or so, then there is surely no evidence that supports this point of view. Changes in the goal of the movement via peripheral feedback require far more time than can be explained by such reflex mechanisms.

It seems clear from the evidence presented in the previous paragraphs that a motor program that produces movement without the involvement of peripheral feedback probably does not exist in human behavior. The problem is not concerned so much with the idea of a program as centrally controlled movement as it is with the stated definition of it, and a change in the definition in order to retain the usefulness of the concept seems necessary. Neurological evidence indicates that both alpha and gamma efferent activity are sent to the musculature, and that they both "cooperate" so that fine reflex adjustments can occur to insure that the movement is carried out as planned. Thus the motor program provides all of the alpha and gamma details necessary for the limbs to reach a certain goal, and feedback is intimately involved in attaining that goal. If the goal needs to be changed because the environment has changed, then the program must run its course for one reaction time (150 msec or so) before a new goal can begin to be achieved. In this case, the reflex mechanisms are active in seeing to it that the old goal—the now "incorrect" goal—is faithfully achieved. This concept can be summarized by defining the motor program *as a set of prestructured alpha and gamma motor commands that, when activated, result in movement oriented toward a given goal, with these movements being unaffected by peripheral feedback indicating that the goal should be changed.*

Notice that there is nothing in this definition that deviates from the original analogy to the computer program. We can imagine that a computer program could have a feedback loop in it that prevents it from attempting to divide by zero, and if the feedback indicated that such a division was going to be attempted, the program could have an instruction that would print out an error message. But all of the instructions to the computer are still prepared in advance, and if the program is consistently reaching a wrong answer (an improper goal), the program cannot be rewritten until it has run its course and the wrong answers are seen.

In summary, the motor program notion, as redefined above, seems essential to account for the evidence indicating that when a movement toward a given goal has been initiated, the movement cannot be changed by feedback information indicating that the goal was inappropriate. Evidence that feedback loop times are far faster than one reaction time do not damage this position at all, as these feedback loops simply ensure that the limbs reach the original, predefined goal, even if that goal is inappropriate. The lack of direct support for the program notion is somewhat disturbing, but abandoning the notion would seem to leave us without an adequate explanation for the control of movements with movement times of less than 150 msec.

C. The Role of Efference Copy

The notion of an "efference copy" has created a great deal of interest recently, but considerable confusion surrounds the idea in part because the term has been used in a variety of ways. From the literature, there are at least three distinct meanings of the concept, and in this section these meanings will be presented so that the position of the schema theory in regard to efference copy will be more clear.

1. The von Holst Position

Von Helmholst (1925) reasoned that in order for accurate visual perception to occur it is essential that the visual system have information about the motor commands sent to the eye musculature. If this information were not present, the organism could not know whether the images that changed on the retina were the result of a moving eye in a stable environment or a stable eye in a moving environment. Later, von Holst (1954) proposed the idea that an efference copy of the instructions sent to the eye muscles was used as a "template" against which to compare and modify the incoming visual signals. If the efference copy indicated whether, or by how much and in what direction, the eye had been moved, the visual information from the retina could be interpreted unambiguously.

Workers in the area of motor control quickly adopted this idea as a potential rival for the motor program notion for movement control, and also to the more traditional feedback control models. The extension to motor control proposed that as the individual initiates the motor commands to the limbs, a copy of the command (the efference copy) is sent to a central storage location. Then, as the movement is being carried out, the incoming proprioceptive signals are compared against the commands that were issued, with any mismatch indicating that an error in responding had occurred. Jones (1971) has referred to this position as the "inflow model" because it depends upon the inflow of proprioceptive feedback to be compared against the efference-copy-based reference of correctness.

There are a number of problems with this formulation, although space limitations do not permit more than a brief mention of them here; see Schmidt (1975a) for a more thorough discussion of these issues. One problem is that the codes for the efference copy and the incoming proprioceptive feedback are in different "languages"; the efference copy is in the "language" of muscle commands, while the proprioceptive feedback is in the "language" of joint motion, skin pressure, and the like. Strictly, how could the two sources of information ever match, just as how could the same idea expressed in French and German ever literally match? It is far too simple to postulate that there is massive recoding throughout the CNS, and that the two sources of information become comparable after they have become recoded. This begs the issue, because now one must specify the theoretical operations underlying this recoding, indicating the hypothetical constructs, postulates, etc., that are required of any theory. Von Holst (1954) must have had something like recoding in mind when he postulated the idea, but not having the operations specified makes the idea untestable.

A second problem with the notion is that it can only indicate to the subject that the movement selected was (or was not) carried out correctly, and it cannot indicate to what extent the goal chosen for the movement was appropriate in meeting the environmental demands. The reason is that the reference of correctness is based upon the commands actually sent, and if the wrong program is chosen, the feedback might match the efference copy (after recoding, of course), and the subject would receive no error information. Thus, this problem concerns the fact that the reference of correctness is tied to the movement actually chosen, and is not related to the achievement of the environmental goal.

2. The Jones Position

Under this view, a copy of the information sent to the musculature is also sent to a storage location in the CNS where the efferent copy is "monitored" centrally, eliminating the delays inherent in the delivery of proprioception. The rationale for this "outflow model" (Jones, 1971) is that if I know where I have told my limbs to go, and I know that my limbs will carry out these orders faithfully, then I know where my limbs are at some time afterward. Thus, the subject is presumed to monitor the motor outflow (the efference copy) to the musculature, and knowing that the efference had reached a certain state provides information about where the limbs are at that point. Also, some writers use this notion (e.g., Angel *et al.*, 1971) to suggest that the subject, via monitoring his own motor outflow, can detect a movement error even before he makes the movement since there is no necessity of waiting until the movement has begun in order to generate feedback as with the previous model.

However, there are a number of problems with the "outflow" model of efference. First, the idea appeared to make a great deal of sense for the perception of the position of the eye (Festinger and Canon, 1965) because of the peculiar properties of the eye-movement system. For example, the eye operates under a nearly constant load, and being able to specify the final location of the eye given the commands provided to the extraocular muscles seemed possible because the loads on the eye are so predictable. However, with the limbs the problem is not so simple because we frequently cannot predict the loads that will be experienced; in such cases, a certain motor outflow may produce any number of final limb positions depending upon the particular loads on the limb. Thus, for perception, there seems to be more necessary (i.e., proprioception) in order that the individual know where his limbs are.

A second problem concerns how the efferent commands are monitored. Although Jones (1971) does not state this in so many words, there is the implication that the efference is monitored against some reference that defines the correct movement. For example, if I wish to move to a particular position, I arouse the reference of correctness (i.e., the reference involved in moving to that position), and then begin to move until the actual efference matches in some way the reference of correctness. When the subject receives the match, he "knows" that he has arrived and he stops moving. One difficulty is in defining how the reference of correctness is learned, and what the variables are that determine its strength; without such statements about the development of this part of the model, the idea remains largely untestable.

3. Efference as a Feedforward Process

A third notion about efference copy is related to the previous two, but is far more general in its statement. Basically, the idea is that when movement commands are sent out to the muscles, the commands are accompanied by other kinds of information that "prepares" the system for the upcoming motor act or for the receipt of sensory information (Teuber, 1964). One example has been mentioned earlier, that dealing with alpha-gamma coactivation. Here, the gamma efferent activity can be thought of a feedforward information that "biases" the muscle spindles in such a way that they can exert fine control over the path of the movement. Such feedforward processes occur throughout the motor system, and these are frequently referred to as efference copy or corollary discharge (Teuber, 1964). Of course, there is no necessity that the efference be a literal copy of the motor commands as with the two previous models, as the gamma efferent activity could take on a form quite different from the alpha activity.

One instance in the schema theory where this version of efference copy is used concerns the generation of the expected sensory consequences. Before the movement begins, the expected proprioception, audition, and vision are aroused and "fed forward" to be later compared with the incoming actual proprioception, audition, and vision in order to detect a movement error. Without this expected feedback state, the resulting feedback could not be interpreted. More basically, the feedforward information seems necessary in order to inform the subject that a program has been executed so that the subject can have information that the feedback that is produced resulted from the carrying out of a program (active movement) versus the movement of the limbs from the environment (passive movement).

There can be little argument with this version of efference because it is so general in its statement. There is strong evidence that such feedforward processes exist, and logical arguments such as are presented in earlier paragraphs indicate that this information is necessary in order that the subject perceive his environment correctly and in order that he detect his own errors in responding. The more precise specification of the generation of the expected sensory consequences in the Schmidt (1975a) schema theory, however, are still open to question, and there are methods available for testing these predictions. The main point here is that such feedforward processes are known to exist, and the postulation of a set of expected sensory consequences is in keeping with the current thinking in neurophysiology.

4. Efference Copy in the Schema Theory

Space in the present chapter does not permit the discussion of the evidence for and against the various efference copy positions, but the evidence is summarized in Schmidt (1975a). Briefly, though, the most important lines of evidence are the deafferentation studies with monkeys (e.g., Taub and Berman, 1968) and the evidence on the rapid correction of errors (e.g., Angel *et al.*, 1971; Megaw, 1972). The deafferentation work indicates that monkeys can learn a bulb-squeeze shock-avoidance response with total loss of feedback from the responding limb, and the implication was that since some form of feedback is needed for learning, it must have been the efference copy that supplied it. Adams (Chapter 4 of this volume) has correctly pointed out that other, nonproprioceptive sources of response information (e.g., vision of the apparatus movements correlated with the bulb-squeeze) might serve as the feedback used to learn the movement. Another possibility is that all that is necessary for learning is information about what motor command was issued (the response specifications in the schema theory) and information about the success of those specifications (the offset of the shock). Either of these explanations can handle the Taub-Berman (1968) findings very well without invoking the Jones (1971) notion of efference copy feedback loops.

The data on rapid error corrections indicate that subjects in two-choice reaction-time tasks sometimes move in the incorrect direction, but often correct their error with latencies (from the initial incorrect move to the beginning of the correction) of about 60 msec, far less than could be explained by peripheral feedback loops. One interpretation (e.g., Angel *et al.*, 1971) is that the subjects monitor their own efferent commands, and detect an error very early in the movement. An alternative explanation, however, is that the subjects anticipate the direction of the move on those error trials, and that the onset of the stimulus light (opposite to their expectations) is the signal which initiates the correction. If so, there is no necessity of postulating the internal monitoring of efference to explain the rapid corrections.

In short, there is no evidence for the first two efference copy models that cannot be handled easily by other explanations, and thus the schema theory position rejects these two views. The third view, that of efference as a series of feedforward mechanisms that "ready" the system for subsequent control, is widely supported by the evidence, and the schema theory is in keeping with this view. Thus, in the schema theory, efference copy has two roles. First, the feeding forward of the expected sensory consequences for later comparison with incoming feedback is fundamentally no different from feeding forward the gamma information to the spindles to alter the reflex influence of subsequent muscle length changes; in both cases errors can be detected, and corrections can be made, although the corrections based upon the expected sensory consequences are considerably slower than those associated with the spindle. Second, the arousal of the expected sensory consequences allows accurate perception of the incoming feedback, and allows the subject to discriminate between active and passive movements.

References

Adams, J.A. (1971). *J. Mot. Behav.* **3**, 111–150.

Angel, R.W., Garland, H., and Fischler, M. (1971). *J. Exp. Psychol.* **89**, 422–424.

Anokhin, P.K. (1969). *In* "A Handbook of Contemporary Soviet Psychology" (M. Cole and I. Maltzman, eds.), pp. 830–856. Basic Books, New York.

Attneave, F. (1957). *J. Exp. Psychol.* **54**, 81–88.

Bartlett, F.C. (1932). "Remembering." Cambridge Univ. Press, London and New York.

Bernstein, N. (1967). "The Co-ordination and Regulation of Movements." Pergamon, Oxford.

Crafts, L.W. (1927). *Arch. Psychol. N.Y.* **14**, No. 91.

Dewhurst, D.J. (1967). *IEEE Trans. Bio-Med. Eng.* **14**, 167–171.

Duncan, C.P. (1958). *J. Exp. Psychol.* **55**, 63–72.

Edmonds, E.M., Mueller, M.R., and Evans, S.H. (1966). *Psychonom. Sci.* **6**, 377–378.

Festinger, I., and Canon, L.K. (1965). *Psychol. Rev.* **72**, 378–384.

Frank, J. (1975). Master's Thesis, University of Waterloo (unpublished).

Granit, R. (1970). "The Basis of Motor Control." Academic Press, New York.

Henry, F.M., and Harrison, J.S. (1961). *Percept. Mot. Skills* **13**, 351–354.

Henry, F.M., and Rogers, D.E. (1960). *Res. Quart.* **31**, 448–458.

Higgins, J.R., and Spaeth, R.K. (1972). *Quest* **17**, 61–69.

Hubbard, A.W. (1960). "Science and Medicine of Exercise and Sports." Harper, New York.

Jones, B. (1971). *Psychol. Bull.* **79**, 386–390.

Jones, B. (1974). *J. Mot. Behav.* **6**, 33–45.

Keele, S.W. (1968). *Psychol. Bull.* **70**, 387–403.

Keele, S.W., and Posner, M.I. (1968). *J. Exp. Psychol.* **77**, 353–363.

Konorski, J. (1967). "Integrative Activity of the Brain." Univ. of Chicago Press, Chicago, Illinois.

Lashley, K.S. (1917). *Amer. J. Physiol.* **43**, 169–194.

Laszlo, J.I. (1967). *Quart. J. Exp. Psychol.* **19**, 344–349.

Laszlo, J.I., and Bairstow, P.J. (1971). *J. Mot. Behav.* **3**, 241–252.

MacNeilage, P.F., and MacNeilage, L.A. (1973). *In* "The Psychophysiology of Thinking" (F.J. McGuigan and R.A. Schoonover, eds.), pp. 417–448. Academic Press, New York.

Megaw, E.D. (1972). *Ergonomics* **15**, 633–643.

Pew, R.W. (1974). *In* "Human Information Processing: Tutorials in Performance and Cognition" (B.H. Kantowitz, ed.). Erlbaum, New York.

Posner, M.I., and Keele, S.W. (1968). *J. Exp. Psychol.* **77**, 353–363.

Posner, M.I., and Keele, S.W. (1970). *J. Exp. Psychol.* **83**, 304–308.

Schmidt, R.A. (1972). *Psychon. Sci.* **27**, 83–85.

Schmidt, R.A. (1974). *Pap., N. Amer. Soc. Psychol. Sport Phys. Act. Nat. Conv., 1974.*

Schmidt, R.A. (1975a). *Psychol. Rev.* **82**, 225–260.

Schmidt, R.A. (1975b). "Motor Skills." Harper, New York.

Schmidt, R.A., and Russell, D.G. (1972). *J. Exp. Psychol.* **96**, 315–320.

Schmidt, R.A., and White, J.L. (1972). *J. Mot. Behav.* **4**, 143–153.

Schmidt, R.A., and Wrisberg, C.A. (1973). *J. Mot. Behav.* **3**, 155–164.

Sears, T.A., and Newsom Davis, J. (1968). *Ann. N.Y. Acad. Sci.* **155**, 183–190.

Slater-Hammel, A.T. (1960). *Res. Quart.* **31**, 217–228.

Smith, J.L. (1969). Doctoral Dissertation, University of Wisconsin, Madison (unpublished).

Sokolov, E.N. (1969). *In* "A Handbook of Contemporary Soviet Psychology" (M. Cole and I. Maltzman, eds.), pp. 671–704. Basic Books, New York.

Sussman, H.M. (1972). *Psychol. Bull.* **77**, 262–272.

Taub, E., and Berman, A.J. (1968). *In* "The Neuropsychology of Spatially Oriented Behavior" (S.J. Freedman, ed.), pp. 172–192. Dorsey, Homewood, Illinois.

Teuber, H.L. (1964). *Acquis. Lang. Monogr. Soc. Res. Child Develop.* **29**, 131–138 (Comment on E.H. Lenneberg's paper: "Speech as a Motor Skill with Special Reference to Nonaphasic Disorders").

von Helmholtz, H. (1925). "Treatise on Physiological Optics" (P.C. Southall, ed. and transl.), 3rd ed., Vol. 3. Op. Soc. Amer., Menasha, Wisconsin.

von Holst, E. (1954). *Brit. J. Anim. Behav.* **2**, 89–94.

Wilson, D.M. (1961). *J. Exp. Biol.* **38**, 471–490.

Spatial Location Cues and Movement Production

David G. Russell

I. Introduction

The production of skilled movement results from the coordination of a number of central processes. The work of Bowditch and Southard (1881) and Woodworth (1899) represents the earliest attempts to model the complexity of skilled performance. Woodworth's (1899) extensive study of movement led him to conclude that accuracy for fast movement depends upon "initial adjustments" of the whole movement, and that slower movements—those of more than 500 msec—used current control. He foresaw then, what was to become known in the 1940s as open- and closed-loop control. Briefly, the closed-loop mode depends upon the knowledge of the course of a movement which arises from the feedback produced by that movement to control it. Under the open-loop mode, movement is considered to occur without reference to peripheral feedback. This latter type is often considered as control by means of a motor program. World War II forced researchers to investigate man as an operator of complex armaments and suggested the value of engineering models.

The two papers published posthumously in Craik's name by Margaret Vince (Craik, 1947, 1948) provided the strongest theoretical framework for open- and closed-loop control. In the first of those two papers, Craik (1947) discussed the role of man as a component of a man-machine system, arguing that the processes of control, and system dynamics required of a man-machine system, apply equally well to man himself. A most important question which Craik did not address concerns the memory component of movement control: What demands do each of these control modes make on memory? Under the traditionally accepted interpretation, open-loop control requires the storage in memory of an infinite number of learned movements in the form of some representation of the motor commands (Henry and Rogers, 1960). Similarly, closed-loop control requires some representation of the sensory consequences of these movements (Adams, 1971). The memory requirements in either case, in terms of the storage and subsequent retrieval, are enormous.

What follows in this chapter is an attempt to raise some of the problems inherent in these traditionally accepted views as they apply to the retention and control of movement. In addition, I shall consider evidence for the coding of movement information and discuss the possibility that movement may be coded in terms of spatial location. Finally, evidence for the utilization of spatial location cues in determining production and control of movement will be provided.

II. Motor Control

A. Motor Programming

Open-loop control implies motor programming in that the motor pattern of innervation is structured prior to release and is not dependent on peripheral feedback. As we shall see, the question of importance concerns the degree to which motor commands are "prestructured."

Central or motor programming was implied in Woodworth's (1889) work, but can be considered to have its empirical origins in one of Lashley's early studies (1917) in which the capacity of a spine-injured patient to reproduce movement was reported. The important conclusion was that "accurate movement of a single joint is possible in the absence of all excitation from the moving organ [p. 193]." If there was no peripheral information to guide the movement, then the only apparent explanation is the central formulation of motor commands. Lashley thus became a proponent of the "centralist" view of motor control, arguing cleverly from the logic of examples which were then unsupported by experimental evidence. In 1951, he proposed that the high rate of movement shown in some skilled performances, such as trills on the piano, forced the conclusion that an effector mechanism can be preset or primed to discharge at a given intensity, or for a given duration independent of any sensory controls (Lashley, 1951). Similar conclusions seem inevitable from Brindley and Merton's work (1960) which suggests that saccadic eye movements are under central or open-loop control (see Festinger and Canon, 1965, for review).

Later research has shown that movement can be performed under conditions of diminished afferent information (Laszlo, 1966, 1967a,b; Laszlo et al., 1974; Provins, 1958). Using a Xylocaine nerve block of the metacarpophalangeal joint, Provins (1958) found a 6% decrement in finger tapping rate over an unanesthetized control condition. Laszlo's studies used the technique of artificially induced ischemia resulting from a nerve compression block[1] originally proposed by Lewis et al. (1931) to produce kinesthetic sense loss. In her paper, Laszlo (1967b) deprived subjects of relevant sensory feedback, including visual, tactile, auditory, and kinesthetic, and found they could still perform finger tapping movements with about the same efficiency as Provin's subjects.

This evidence, together with that of nonhuman research findings of Nottebohm (1970) with birdsongs, Wilson (1961, 1964) with locust's flight patterns, and Taub and Berman (1968) with surgically deafferented monkeys, seems to force the conclusion that the movement may occur as the result of centrally stored neural commands which are "structured before the movement begins and allows the entire movement to be carried out uninfluenced by peripheral feedback [Keele, 1968, p. 387]."

The idea of motor programming has been implied or expounded in the work of others, notably Pew (1966), Roy (1973), and Schmidt and Russell (1972). Pew (1966) used a compensatory tracking task requiring alternate key pressing with right and left hands to keep a dot centered on a screen and found evidence for open-loop control. Some subject's appeared to respond with rapid series of alternations making no apparent corrections until the error exceeded some values, at which time adjustive feedback-controlled movements appeared to be made to correct the drift.

Motor programming, or open-loop control, as evidenced above, is exemplified in the "memory drum" theory of Henry and Rogers (1960). The theory postulates the storage of neural commands which, upon their elicitation, are transmitted to the appropriate muscles in the correct temporal sequence to produce the movement. Inherent in programming theory is the notion that, at most, some representation of the neural commands that produce the movement is stored in memory and, at least, the general movement pattern for each movement is retained in memory. This representation could be used as the basis for the generation of the motor commands. The latter alternative will be discussed in greater detail when the question of the "spontaneous" generation of

---

[1] For details of the procedures for the nerve compression block technique refer to Laszlo and Bairstow (1971b).

movement is reviewed. For example, Pew's study (1966) with its extended practice of several months could be interpreted as support for the retention of the open-loop phase by some subjects.

B. Closed-Loop Control

In movements longer than feedback processing time, there occurs the potential for using afferent information in the ongoing control of movement. Chernikoff and Taylor (1952) measured kinesthetic reaction time as the interval from the moment of release of a horizontally supported relaxed arm until the onset of deceleration as the subject reacted to arrest the downward movement of his limb. This reaction time ranged from 119 to 129 msec. Higgins and Angel (1970), using similar methodology, found a kinesthetic reaction time of between 108 and 169 msec. Keele and Posner (1968) estimate the minimum time to receive and act upon visual information to be between 190 and 260 msec. The critical duration below which feedback control can occur, therefore, seems to be about 150 msec (Schmidt, 1972). Further, Schmidt and Russell (1972) have shown that movement time seems to be the major determiner of whether a movement is preprogrammed or whether it is feedback dependent. Movements of approximately 160 msec showed little reliance, and those of about 650 msec much reliance, on peripheral feedback.

The idea of feedback involvement in motor control is not new. James (1890) proposed that peripheral feedback from one segment of a movement "triggers" the next; and postulated a "reflex chaining hypothesis." The same idea is also seen in the peripheral theory of language. Washburn (1916) proposed "successive motor systems" in which the "stimulus furnished by the actual performance of the criterion movements is required to bring about other movements [p. 11]." Bartlett (1948), however, was more specific when he suggested that a response is "not merely set off by a receptor function, but is guided by it [p. 31]," thus inferring feedback control.

A direct and cohesive determination of the role of feedback in movement control became possible with the introduction of engineering concepts to experimental psychology, largely through the work of Craik (1947, 1948). These papers stem primarily from his philosophical treatise (Craik, 1943) on an approach to investigating man's performance. In the two later papers Craik developed the proposition that "the human operator behaves basically as an intermittent correction servo [Craik, 1947, p. 56]." Feedback utilization in motor control has also led to the development of a number of closed-loop models of human behavior (Adams, 1961, 1968, 1971; Chase, 1965a,b; Fairbanks, 1954; Laszlo and Bairstow, 1971a; von Holst, 1954; Welford, 1960).

Adams (1971, p. 120) points out that a closed-loop theory must be error-centered, and have a "reference mechanism against which feedback from the response is compared for detection of error. . . ." Thus, the closed-loop control of learned movements requires that the sensory consequences of the present response be compared with some representation of the desired response to check its accuracy in achieving its specified goal. Implicit in this control mode, then, are three basic processes: the transmission and reception of feedback from the ongoing response by some comparator; detection of any error in the ongoing response resulting from the comparison of that feedback with some representation of the required movements; and the generation and execution of subsequent corrective movement on the basis of the detected error. In Adams' (1971) theory, in particular, the representation of the sensory consequences of past successful responses is a function of the subject's knowledge of previous performance.

Craik (1948) himself, while arguing for the intermittency of apparently continous responses, conceded that another mode of control was necessary to explain the type of behavior exhibited by telegraph operators (e.g., Bryan and Harter, 1899), who transmit series of letters while apparently paying no attention to the movements. It was apparent, Craik (1948) argued, that complex patterns could be established which could be triggered as a whole (cf. Woodworth, 1899); in other words, that there are two types of control: open- and closed-loop.

While both these theories are well entrenched in motor behavior, I suspect that both Craik and Woodworth would have agreed with Keele (1968) when he said in a trivial sense that all movements are programmed. The point being, of course, that irrespective of whether a movement, in the traditional view, is open- or closed-loop controlled, at a "micro" level it must be preprogrammed. Short-duration, corrective movements, as required by closed-loop control, must be determined predictively. That is, the corrective movement must be produced so that the error detected at t_1 and the error predicted for t_2, $(t_1 + \Delta t)$ must be accounted for and corrected, Δt being the time for the reception of error information to the time when the corrective movement is effected. The commands that correct error, therefore, must be to a position which the system predicts will be correct at t_2. The argument, therefore, is not open- or closed-loop control, but rather the accuracy of predicted position. This point will be taken up later.

C. Implications of Control Mode for Motor Memory

The implications for motor memory of both open- and closed-loop theories can be seen in Stelmach's (1974) argument in equating retention with "persistence of habit." He points out that what is encoded in memory has to be determined before we can decide what is maintained. What must be encoded into memory, and therefore basic to the operation of both programmed and closed-loop control modes, is some representation of past successful responses. In the case of programmed control, the representation is of the efferent commands which lead to the movement (Henry and Rogers, 1960). In closed-loop control, the representation is of the afferent information which has arisen from successful responses which provide a reference level, or perceptual trace (Adams, 1971) for movement control. This point is important because it implies that a representation of every learned movement, in terms of either the afferent or efferent component, is required for production and control.

The magnitude of this problem can be seen in serially ordered behavior. Lashley (1951), in his classic paper, "The Problem of Serial Order in Behavior," argues that the motor elements in speech used to express meaning have some organization imposed upon them. This imposition is from the idea the individual wishes to communicate on the words used. The words used determine the phonemes, and the order in which they are formulated. However, if the durations of the articulatory movements are such that ongoing closed-loop control is not possible, then patterns of neural activity must be either recovered from storage or generated afresh from nonspecific movement information for each phoneme.

The actual process of serial ordering of speech can be seen as phoneme neural commands determined by the "higher order structure of the language [MacNeilage, 1970, p. 183]." Such workers in speech physiology as Halle (1964), Liberman *et al.* (1967), and Lindblom (1963) are of the opinion that the production of speech is the result of the motor programming of phonemes in the Henry and Rogers (1960) sense. That is, for every phoneme, there is in memory a set of motor commands. However, the number of required sets of phoneme commands is far in excess of the number of phonemes in the English language. MacNeilage and DeClerk (1969) demonstrated that the pattern of innervation of a given phoneme is influenced by the identity of adjacent phonemes. Thus, it would be a question not of the number of phonemes the neural commands of which must be stored, but rather of the number of allophones[2] which must be stored, in order that the English language be spoken. MacNeilage and DeClerk (1969) used as their basic technique electromyographic (EMG) recordings of muscular involvement in the production of given vowels under conditions which varied preceding and following consonant phonemes. By analyzing cinefluoroscopic records they confirmed the earlier finding of Kozhevnikov and Chistovich (1965) that the terminal position of the tongue was relatively invariant.

Thus, MacNeilage and DeClerk's (1969) results showed relatively constant terminations of articulatory components to be associated with EMG activity which varied according to the identity of the adjacent phoneme. MacNeilage

---

[2] The term "allophone" refers to any of the variants making up a single phoneme.

(1970), basing his calculations on those of Denes (1963) concerning the statistics of spoken English, estimated the total number of stored allophones required for speaking at a given rate to be at least 40,000. When stress variations are considered, the number is considered to be over 100,000. The selection and accession of the appropriate program for a series of phonemes which constitute a given utterance, while conceivable, seems rather cumbersome. Of course, speech is not the only type of movement behavior which raises this problem. It is essentially the same for the production and control of typing, writing, playing the piano and other musical instruments, and to some extent all learned movements. Further, it applies whether programmed or closed-loop control is used. In the latter case, it requires the availability of some reference against which to assess the ongoing response. This calls for the same number of references for closed-loop control as programming requires neural pattern representations. If it seems unparsimonious to store the actual pattern of neural innervations or the sensory consequences of each learned movement as the basis for control, is there an alternative?

III. Coding and the Availability of Movement Cues

The question here is, Which movement cues are suitable for the generation and control of movement? The evidence for the coding of movement information follows, and, as will be shown, location appears to be the most precisely codable.

While movement information can obviously be derived from exteroceptive sources such as vision and audition, the following discussion is concerned with kinesthetic cues. There is evidence for the existence of receptors for a number of dimensions of kinesthesis such as position, amplitude and velocity (Marteniuk *et al.*, 1972), acceleration (Fuchs, 1962), and force (Russell and Marteniuk, 1974). Of these, most of the considerable evidence has accrued for position. That position sense is a legitimate dimension of the kinesthetic modality is derived from both physiological and behavioral investigations. Of the physiological studies, Mountcastle and Powell (1959), for example, showed a "rather precise relation of the activity of a cortical neuron to the angle of the joint [p. 128]." Boyd and Roberts (1953), studying the knee joint of the cat, demonstrated a characteristic discharge frequency of receptors for particular positions and rates of movement. Further, Gardner (1966) suggests that when a joint is at rest, the slowly adapting spray endings most sensitive at that position continue to discharge for some time. Finally, Mountcastle *et al.* (1963) manipulated the knee joints of monkeys and recorded the firing rates of cells in the thalamic ventrobasal nuclei, together with the angles of the joints which drive these cells. They found that some neurons fire maximally when the limb is fully extended, and others when it is fully flexed. Summarizing the evidence regarding positional receptors, Smith (1969, p. 34) concluded:

1. Receptors fire at different frequencies for a specific joint angle, regardless of the speed or direction from which the position was approached.
2. Receptors adapt slowly and often a single unit has a different adaptation rate for each joint angle.
3. More receptors are responsive to a limited range of the total joint action.

This summary of Smith's is based on passive movement. Jones (1974) considers such evidence irrelevant to theories of skill which must be concerned with only voluntary movement. However, it should be pointed out that such studies of passive movement have much to say about the mechanisms underlying the encoding of movement cues, in that they provide the afferent information on the basis of which this encoding occurs. Certainly there is adequate evidence for the perception and, therefore, the potential for the central coding of position. However, the mere existence of physiological evidence for the transduction of limb position is not in itself sufficient, for its central storage.

While it is apparent that there are receptors capable of accurately indicating limb position, there is much behavioral evidence which adds to the argument that location is a potential source of movement control information. Marteniuk and Roy (1972a,b) showed that location cues seem to provide the major source of codable information for movement reproduction.

Some confusion seems to exist in numerous studies regarding the type of sensory information under consideration. For example, studies of both active movement (Cohen, 1958; Marteniuk, 1971; Wood, 1969), and of passive movement (Cleghorn and Darcus, 1952; Laidlaw and Hamilton, 1937) were probably more concerned with location, than with movement per se. Linear positioning, and lever rotation tasks are often used in the investigation of the psychophysics of kinesthesis (Marteniuk, 1971; Shields, 1970; Wood, 1969), and short-term motor memory (Adams and Dijkstra, 1966; Stelmach, 1969, 1970; Williams et al., 1969). The greatest confusion has occurred from the failure to differentiate the extent of a movement (distance) and its end point (location). For example Brown et al. (1948) stated the purpose of their study to be the accuracy of positioning. Their instructions asked subjects to "concentrate on the distance between these two . . . points [p. 171]." Although not explicitly stated, their instructions assumed that subjects were coding distance rather than location. More recent investigators have similarly confused the two types of cues. For example, some have assumed or stated the distance as the appropriate cue for reproduction (Marteniuk, 1971; Stelmach and Wilson, 1970), and others, position (Posner and Konick, 1966; Stelmach, 1969).

Posner (1967) recognized the need to experimentally differentiate distance and location cues which he attempted to accomplish by making location an unreliable cue for one of his experimental groups, (distance), while the other group, (location), had both distance and location cues available. Essentially, the task required subjects to rotate a handle in one box, and then to reproduce it in another, adjacent box. To assess the accuracy of the reproduction in the distance condition, the subject rotated the lever in the first box either 20°, 40°, 60°, 70°, 80°, or 90° for the standard movement, and then attempted to reproduce that extent from a different starting position in the second box. In the location condition, the subject reproduced, in the second box, the movement made in the first, from the same starting position to the same location as the standard. There were no significant differences between these two conditions. There are some fundamental problems concerning the foregoing results. First, one of the conditions involved both distance and location, while the other had distance cues available. The failure of the experimental manipulation to produce any difference could be explained by subjects ignoring the location cues and utilizing the common distance cues. This would mean that distance cues are more precisely codable than location cues. This seems unlikely in view of the findings of Keele and Ells (1972) and Marteniuk and Roy (1972b), who showed location more precisely codable than distance. Second, the location group was not called on to reproduce the precise end point of the standard movement because the reproduction movement was performed on a different lever in a different box. As Corrigan and Brogden's (1949) findings show, there is differential accuracy in movement to different locations relative to the body.

Marteniuk et al. (1972) further investigated the question of the codability of location and distance cues. They attempted to make subjects rely on either distance or location cues. Their results suggested that recall of distance resulted in greater error. They concluded that movement or distance information per se was not as precisely codable as location information. Marteniuk and Roy (1972b) extended this line of investigation by determining what influence random, passively induced movements would have on the codability of location cues. If distance per se cannot be encoded, the random movements imposed during presentation of the standard should have no effect on the accuracy of reproduction. Their result suggested quite strongly that for linear positioning at least, "location cues provide a major source of codable information for movement reproduction" (Marteniuk and Roy, 1972b, p. 477) and that distance information is not very precise, or is even uncodable, when it is the only information available. Keele and Ells (1972) support this contention using a task similar to Posner's study (1967). They investigated the roles of location, distance plus location, and tension, concluding that of these, the only cue which remained stable over their manipulations was location. They suggest that subjects may have relied more on location cues than on distance or tension cues because the task required the movement of only one joint. Even so, there was some evidence for the use of distance cues in the reproduction of short movements.

However, Keele and Ells (1972) rightly point out distance cues may be derived from location information. Smith (1969) and Skoglund (1956) would tend to agree with these general findings in that their literature reviews failed to identify receptors subservient to movement extent, but did for velocity, acceleration and direction.

Collectively, this evidence suggests that location is codable in memory; the physiological evidence shows that there are sensory receptors which subserve limb position, and the behavioral evidence shows that such information transmitted from these receptors can be centrally coded. The question that has not been answered with any clarity is: How is limb position encoded as location? The physiological evidence for position receptors is for joint angle. As Keele and Ells (1972) imply, determining location from the angle of a single joint is relatively simple, but it becomes increasingly complex as more joints are used. It seems apparent, intuitively at least, that the sensory information from receptors subservient to joint angle is insufficient to permit the direct coding of spatial location.[3] Lashley (1951) has suggested a "space coordinate" system (p. 126)—reference systems which permit us to remember our location with reference to other locations. For example, we can find a number of ways home from work, and equally importantly from work to home, given that we know where we are and its relationship to where we wish to go. In terms of movement, Lashley (1951, p. 126) states of these space coordinate systems:

> Their influences pervade the motor system so that every gross movement of limbs or body is made with reference to the space system. The perceptions from the distance receptors, vision, hearing, and touch, are also constantly modified and referred to the same space co-ordinates. The stimulus is *there*, in a definite place; it has definite relation to the position of the body, and it shifts with respect to the sense organ, but not with respect to the general orientation, with changes in body posture . . . such space characters provide a possible basis for some serial actions. . . .

There is obvious potential for such a system as Lashley suggests in the coding of spatial location. It is possible that there is a transformation to spatial location from joint angle information, and that it is the result of this transformation, as we shall see, on which motor control may be based.

IV. Spatial Location and Movement Control

The evidence presented above shows that sensory information from limb position receptors is available, and that spatial location is encoded in memory on

---

[3] I shall henceforth use *spatial location*. That term implies the coding of a point in space, not just joint angle which is implied by location because the sensory information from which it is derived references joint angle.

the basis of this and other, exteroceptive (e.g., visual), information. This latter transformation from limb position to spatial location, or to a space coordinate reference, as Lashley (1951) suggests, has important consequences for movement control, in that it frees the motor system from reliance on either stored motor commands, or sensory consequences from movement reproduction and control. That is, given the desired location encoded in memory, the motor system may be able to reduce the discrepancy between current and desired location.

This introduces the potential for a degree of plasticity of movement generation. That is, it is possible that spatial location information is the only specific, stored information required to generate novel movements, and to reproduce learned movements in that the subject "generates afresh" (MacNeilage and MacNeilage, 1973, p. 434) the neural commands required to achieve the desired spatial location. Such a procedure seems necessary in the production of speech. The articulation of any utterance requires movement of the articulators to the positions required for its component phonemes. The production of the first phoneme of the utterance may require movement of the articulators to the location specific to that phoneme from virtually any other position. That initial movement is contingent on prespeech position has been shown by MacNeilage and DeClerk (1969). MacNeilage (1970) suggests that perfectly intelligible speech can occur as a result of the spontaneous reorganization of the movement pattern of the tongue and lips, as in the case of the teeth-clenching pipesmoker.

The necessity of having an alternative to the generation and control of speech by stored motor commands, is seen in this quote from MacNeilage (1970, p. 184).

> . . . it is difficult to believe that a speech production system based on the storage of discrete movement patterns could make such a spontaneous adjustment by immediately producing a new set of commands.

Note that this type of system requires that the encoding in memory of the terminal location of movement must be independent of the movement(s) associated with its encoding. This independence refers to the transformation from sensory information to a space coordinate such as was discussed in the previous section. This transformation makes the spatial location of a position available independently of the movements associated with its encoding in memory. As we shall see later, there is some evidence for the differentiation of terminal location from its associated movements in linear positioning (Marteniuk and Roy, 1972a,b) lever rotation (Laabs, 1973) as well as two-dimensional movement (Russell, 1974).

The independent encoding of spatial location is the premise upon which the MacNeilage target hypothesis is based. Working within the framework of the motor control of speech, MacNeilage (1973) has proposed a system for the production and control of articulation in which the essential feature is the terminal location, or target, of the various components of the articulatory mechanism. This hypothetical system forms the basis of the target hypothesis and forms a major alternative to the contention that each phoneme is produced from invariant motor commands. In essence, MacNeilage (1970) has proposed that the location of the target is coded in memory, and that it may be regarded as a specification of a point within the space coordinate system. The hypotheses proposes that this coded location information is the information required by a motor system which can produce a response to the target. This, according to MacNeilage and MacNeilage (1973), permits movements to be "generated afresh—each time they are required by a mechanism . . . which has the potential for creativity" (p. 434). Note that they do not consider articulatory movement to be the result of stored patterns of neural activity (cf. Halle, 1964; Liberman *et al.*, 1967; Lindblom, 1963; Wickelgren, 1969), but rather to be spontaneously generated on the basis of target specifications of the utterance required. This clear implication of the spontaneous production of apparently learned movement is a radical departure from the belief that either the motor commands (Henry and Rogers, 1960), or the sensory consequences of the movement to be produced (Adams, 1971), are stored for accurate movement production.

Sussman (1972) states that only a system that is constantly informed of the moment-to-moment position and movement rate of a component can accomplish the high degree of movement control required in speech. A motor system informed of current spatial location and a knowledge of desired spatial location can, therefore, act to reduce the discrepancy between the two. In the same paper, Sussman suggests such a system based on gamma motor control. Clearly, if such a system is capable of controlling the rapid, and serially ordered movements required for speech, a similar system has the potential for the control of nonspeech movement; probably even more so because, whereas the accoustical consequences of speech movements are not available until after the completion of those movements (particularly early in practice), the visual consequences of nonspeech movement are often available concurrently with the movement. When concurrent visual information is not available, the system should, theoretically, be at no more of a disadvantage than the highly successful motor system for speech. However, there should be some caution expressed in accepting this position. Jones (1974) notes that the absence of visual information decreases efficiency in learning movements. However, as suggested above, exteroceptive information, especially visual, may make a major contribution to the coding of spatial location. Further, the studies cited by Jones regarded tasks in which all components of the criterion movements were within visual range. Consequently, such objections could not apply to components of movements which do not occur within the visual range.

Earlier in this discussion I argued that, in essence, there is no real difference between closed-loop and open-loop control, quoting Keele's statement (1968), that in a trivial sense all movements are motor programmed. It may be in a not-so-trivial sense that all movements are preprogrammed. As pointed out earlier, even in closed-loop control, e.g., tracking, the movement commands produced at time, t_1, must take account of current error plus the error which, it is predicted, will occur at time, $t_1 + \Delta t$, or t_2. This prediction, in a very real sense, may be based on the prediction of spatial location of the limb at t_2 in relation to the desired terminal position for that movement. Thus, whether thought of in terms of the small adjustive movements in tracking the desired movement path to the terminal point, or of the overall reduction in discrepancy between the starting location and the desired terminal point, the motor system may very well be simply operating to reduce the discrepancy between actual and desired spatial location. In the one case, the desired location is predicted, in the other it is stored, encoded in memory from past movements, not as part of these movements, but independent of them.

V. Evidence

For spatial location to be a viable alternative to the stored neural commands or their sensory consequences in the production and control of movement, two things must be shown. First, the spatial location is accessible in memory independently of any movement(s) associated with its storage, and second, that movement to that location can be produced from starting positions other than that from which the spatial location was coded.

Let us return for a moment to the MacNeilage target hypotheses. Recall that the two main features of that hypothesis are the storage of locations specific to particular phonemes, and the capability given that target information, to generate movements to those targets.

Marteniuk and Roy (1972b) and Laabs (1973) have shown that a given location can be reproduced when the recall starting position differs from that of the initial movement. It should be pointed out that movements in these studies are unidimensional in that the path of the movement is restricted by the track on which the lever is mounted. Nevertheless, the findings of the two studies support the contention that spatial location is available independently of the movement extents associated with its storage. Of course, it would be more convincing if the same results could be obtained where the task provides the potential for directional, as well as amplitude, error. Further, if these results can be obtained, there are implications for motor control as well. Consider the following requirements. If the subject makes movements from one or more starting positions to a specific location (initial movements), and then is later asked to move to that same location (criterion movement) from a different starting position, accurate reproduction of the criterion location would be based on the *location information* because no specific movement extent information would be available to the subjects. The only element common to both initial and criterion movements would be the end point on location. This would mean not only that the criterion location was accessible in memory independently of the movement(s) associated with its storage, but also that it must have been the basis of the production and control of the criterion movement.

The actual task (Russell, 1974) involved moving a right-hand-held pencil from a fixed starting point a distance of 16.2 cm to a short-duration dot of light which served as the target. Both the presentation of the target and the movement occurred in the dark. There were 30 criterion trials with knowledge of results after each. Subjects performed under one of five conditions immediately before the criterion movement. Relevant in the present context are three conditions. Group I moved from six randomly assigned, noncriterion starting points to the target for a total of 60 movements. Thus, proprioceptive and visual information about the target was available since the initial starting positions were other than that of the criterion movement. Group II made their 60 initial movements from the criterion starting position and, therefore, had both specific movement extent and target information. Group III was a control condition in which no initial movements were given. Using as the dependent measure the absolute deviation of the termination of the criterion movement from the target (radial error), the results showed that the accuracy of reproduction of the target by subjects in both experimental conditions (groups I and II) was superior to that of the control. Also, groups I and II did not differ reliably in terms of their radial error. The findings concerning group I may be taken as support for the contention that spatial location can be encoded in memory, and that the movement to this spatial location was produced and controlled on the basis of the location information in the absence of movement information per se. While group II had both movement and location information, group I had only location information. Further, unlike Laabs (1973) and Marteniuk and Roy (1972b), the direction of the criterion movement for group I was novel to the subjects in that condition. Thus, subjects in the Russell study (1974) had even less information on which to base the production of the movement to the target: The criterion movement was produced on the basis of spatial location information derived from visual and proprioceptive information.

The argument may be made that subjects in group I had sufficient location information on which to formulate the appropriate neural commands, or of their sensory consequences and that this caused performance to improve rapidly over two or three trials, to the level of group II and that the results, averaged over trials, reflects nothing other than a ceiling effect. However, a further analysis of trial I performance yielded similar results. A subsequent study by Russell and Simon (1974) similarly showed no significant difference between conditions comparable to groups I and II in Russell's study (1974) on the first criterion trial and performance on both these conditions was superior to control conditions.

These results may be interpreted in terms of the implications for motor control. That is, in the absence of specific movement information, including directional information, subjects were capable of reducing the discrepancy between a novel starting position and a centrally coded spatial location, implying that neither the neural commands nor the sensory consequences of the criterion moved were necessary for the production and control of accurate movement to a target.

VI. Implications

In the previous section evidence was presented which suggests that movement may be produced and controlled on the basis of little other than stored spatial location information. If this is so, there must exist some central response organization system that can operate to reduce the discrepancy between currently perceived location and desired location which is either centrally stored or predicted. The exact nature of a suitable mechanism, while of obvious importance, is not essential to the proposed theoretical response organization system. The existence of such a system is derived from evidence of linear positioning, both with and without directional constraints and has been discussed in the previous section. But what of more complex movements?

Take, for example, a baseball pitcher. There is a position in space relative to his body at which the ball must be released if the ball is to go where he wishes. But even before this point there are similar positions which he has learned from thousands of pitches that bring him to the point of release—the point at which his glove hand and pitching hand meet in the preparatory movement, the point at which they part, the end of the backswing of his pitching hand and elbow, the point at which the elbow "waits" for the hand to accelerate past it to deliver the ball. This is, of course, grossly oversimplified. But if spatial location can be the basis of movement production and control, then such movements may occur as the result of a central response organization system reducing the discrepancy between the current locations of the body components, and the next series of desired spatial locations. The important difference between this and the memory requirements of traditionally viewed programmed and closed-loop control is that these spatial locations, rather than the neural commands or their sensory consequences, would be stored. What is happening under the proposed control system is that the response organization system produced, on the basis of the spatial location reference requirements, a set of neural commands which, it predicts, will reduce the discrepancy between initial and desired location. This does not preclude the possibility of the requirement imposed upon motor systems by Sussman (1972) that moment-to-moment corrections can be made on the basis of information regarding the actual current and the desired track to the ultimate spatial location for that movement. In moment-to-moment correction, the system is saying, in effect, I am now here, but by the time I generate this corrective movement, inertia will have carried me to there. Therefore, the corrective movement must take me to where I predict I should be by the time it is organized and effected. The sum of these "corrective movements" will lead ultimately to the desired spatial location for the whole movement. The important point is that the movement is not performed on the basis of stored movement information per se, but on the basis of stored, or predicted spatial locations. Thus, to paraphrase Keele (1968) once again, in a not so trivial sense, all movements are motor programmed, if by motor programmed is meant the production of patterns of neural innervation which will take body components to desired spatial locations.

This, then, brings us full circle to Woodworth's (1899) contention that accuracy for fast movements depends upon "initial adjustments" which are adjustments of the whole movement occurring at the outset of the movement, and slower movements use current control; this current control can be thought of as the result of on-line adjustive movements to predicted locations which keep the movement directed toward a desired spatial location.

VII. Summary

In this chapter I have attempted to show some deficiencies in trying to account for the production and control of movement under the traditionally accepted view of programmed and closed-loop control which are based on stored information of the neural commands to muscles (e.g., Henry and Rogers, 1960) or their sensory consequences (e.g., Adams, 1971). An alternative is suggested which is based on two assumptions: First, that spatial location is a transformation of sensory information not necessarily stored in terms of the actual afferent information. A space coordinate reference system such as Lashley (1951) has suggested is potentially suitable for the product of such a notion. And, second, that movement production and control may be based upon this spatial location information, centrally stored, or predicted, given a knowledge of current location. The production and control would be achieved by some response organization system which is capable of generating neural commands to take body components to desired spatial locations. This means that movement may be generated on the basis of stored spatial location rather than specific movement information, overcoming the problems inherent in the storage and access of movement information specific to every action.

Acknowledgments

The preparation of this chapter was supported in part by the State of Illinois Department of Mental Health to the Motor and Leisure Behavior Research Laboratory of the Children's

Research Center, University of Illinois, via the Adler Zone Center, Champaign, Illinois, and in part by URG funds provided by the University of Queensland, St. Lucia, Queensland, Australia.

The author gratefully acknowledges the comments on an earlier draft of this chapter of Dr. Bill Jones and Dr. Judith Laszlo.

References

Adams, J.A. (1961). *Psychol. Bull.* **58**, 55–79.

Adams, J.A. (1968). *Psychol. Bull.* **70**, 486–504.

Adams, J.A. (1971). *J. Mot. Behav.* **3**, 111–149.

Adams, J.A., and Dijkstra, S. (1966). *J. Exp. Psychol.* **71**, 314–318.

Bartlett, F.C. (1948). *Occup. Psychol.* **22**, 31–38.

Bowditch, H.P., and Southard, W.F. (1881). *J. Physiol. (London)* **3**, 232–245.

Boyd, I.A., and Roberts, T.M. (1953). *J. Physiol. (London)* **1**, 122–138.

Brindley, G.S., and Merton, P.A. (1960). *J. Physiol. (London)* **153**, 127–130.

Brown, J.S., Knauft, E.B., and Rosenbaum, G. (1948). *Amer. J. Psychol.* **61**, 167–182.

Bryan, W.L., and Harter, N. (1899). *Psychol. Rev.* **6**, 345–375.

Chase, R.A. (1965a). *J. Nerv. Ment. Dis.* **140**, 239–251.

Chase, R.A. (1965b). *J. Nerv. Ment. Dis.* **140**, 334–350.

Chernikoff, R., and Taylor, F.V. (1952). *J. Exp. Psychol.* **43**, 1–8.

Cleghorn, T.E., and Darcus, H.D. (1952). *Quart. J. Exp. Psychol.* **4**, 66–77.

Cohen, L.A. (1958). *J. Neurophysiol.* **21**, 550–562.

Corrigan, R.E., and Brogden, W.J. (1949). *Amer. J. Psychol.* **62**, 90–98.

Craik, K.J.W. (1943). "The Nature of Explanation." Cambridge Univ. Press, London and New York.

Craik, K.J.W. (1947). *Brit. J. Psychol.* **38**, 56–61.

Craik, K.J.W. (1948). *Brit. J. Psychol.* **38**, 142–148.

Denes, P.M. (1963). *J. Acoust. Soc. Amer.* **35**, 892–904.

Fairbanks, G. (1954). *J. Speech Hear. Disabil.* **19**, 133–139.

Festinger, L., and Canon, L.K. (1965). *Psychol. Rev.* **72**, 373–384.

Fuchs, A.H. (1962). *J. Exp. Psychol.* **63**, 177–182.

Gardner, E. (1967). *Myotatic, Kinesthetic Vestibular Mech., Ciba Found. Symp.* pp. 56–76.

Gibbs, C.B. (1954). *Brit. J. Psychol.* **45**, 24–39.

Halle, M. (1964). *In* "The Structure of Language" (J.A. Fodor and J.J. Katz, eds.), pp. 324–333. Prentice-Hall, Englewood Cliffs, New Jersey.

Henry, F.M., and Rogers, D.E. (1960). *Res. Quart.* **31**, 448–458.

Higgins, J.R., and Angel, R.W. (1970). *J. Exp. Psychol.* **84**, 412–416.

James, W. (1890). "Principles of Psychology." Holt, New York.

Jones, B. (1974). *J. Mot. Behav.* **6**, 33–45.

Keele, S.W. (1968). *Psychol. Bull.* **70**, 387–403.

Keele, S.W., and Ells, J.G. (1972). *J. Mot. Behav.* **4**, 127–134.

Keele, S.W., and Posner, M.I. (1968). *J. Exp. Psychol.* **77**, 155–158.

Kozhevnikov, V.A., and Chistovich, L.A. (1965). "Rech: Artikulatsiya i Vospriyatiye" *(Speech: Articulation and Perception).* Nauka, Moscow (translation: JRRS No. 30543. U.S. Dep. of Commerce, Washington, D.C.).

Laabs, G.J. (1973). *J. Exp. Psychol.* **100**, 168–177.

Laidlaw, R.W., and Hamilton, M.M. (1937). *Bull. Neurol. Inst. New York* **6**, 145–153.

Lashley, K.S. (1917). *Amer. J. Physiol.* **43**, 169–194.

Lashley, K.S. (1951). *In* "Cerebral Mechanisms of Behavior" (L.A. Jeffress, ed.), pp. 112–136. Wiley, New York.

Laszlo, J.I. (1966). *Quart. J. Exp. Psychol.* **18**, 1–8.

Laszlo, J.I. (1967a). *Physiol. & Behav.* **2**, 359–365.

Laszlo, J.I. (1967b). *Quart. J. Exp. Psychol.* **19**, 344–349.

Laszlo, J.I., and Bairstow, P.J. (1971a). *J. Mot. Behav.* **3**, 241–252.

Laszlo, J.I., and Bairstow, P.J. (1971b). *J. Mot. Behav.* **3**, 313–317.

Laszlo, J.I., Bairstow P., and Russell, D.G. (1974). *Pro. Aust. Psychol. Soc.* **5**, 87 (abstr.).

Lewis, T., Pickering, G.W., and Rothschild, P. (1931). *Heart* **16**, 1.

Liberman, A.M., Cooper, F.S., Shankweiler, D.P., and Studdert-Kennedy, M.G. (1967). *Psychol. Rev.* **74**, 431–461.

Lindbolm, B.E. (1963). *J. Acoust. Soc. Amer.* **35**, 1773–1781.

MacNeilage, P.F. (1970). *Psychol. Rev.* **77**, 182–196.

MacNeilage, P.F. (1973). *In* "Speech and Cortical Functioning" (J.H. Gilbert, ed.), pp. 1–72. Academic Press, New York.

MacNeilage, P.F., and DeClerk, J.G. (1969). *J. Acoust. Soc. Amer.* **45**, 1217–1233.

MacNeilage, P.F., and MacNeilage, L.A. (1973). *In* "The Psychophysiology of Thinking" (F.J. McGuigan and R.A. Schoonover, eds.), pp. 417–448. Academic Press, New York.

Marteniuk, R.G. (1971). *J. Mot. Behav.* **3**, 69–77.

Marteniuk, R.G., and Roy, E.A. (1972a). *In* "Psychomotor Learning and Sports Psychology" (I.D. Williams and L.A. Wankel, eds.), pp. 122–130. Amateur Fitness and Sports Directorate, Ottawa, Canada.

Marteniuk, R.G., and Roy, E.A. (1972b). *Acta Psychol.* **36**, 471–479.

Marteniuk, R.G., Shields, K.W.D., and Campbell, S. (1972). *Percept. Mot. Skills* **35**, 51–58.

Mountcastle, V.B., and Powell, T.P.S. (1959). *Johns Hopkins Med. Bull.* **108**, 173–200.

Mountcastle, V.B., Poggio, C.F., and Werner, C. (1963). *J. Exp. Psychol.* **75**, 103–107.

Nottebohm, F. (1970). *Science* **167**, 950–956.

Pew, R.W. (1966). *J. Exp. Psychol.* **71**, 764–771.

Posner, M.I. (1967). *J. Exp. Psychol.* **75**, 103–107.

Posner, M.I., and Konick, A.F. (1966). *Organized Behav. Hum. Performance* **1**, 71–86.

Provins, K.A. (1958). *J. Physiol. (London)* **143**, 55–67.

Roy, E.A. (1973). Master's Thesis, University of British Columbia (unpublished).

Russell, D.G. (1974). Doctoral Dissertation, The University of Michigan, Ann Arbor.

Russell, D.G., and Marteniuk, R.G. (1975). *Percept. & Psychophys.* **16**, 443–448.

Russell, D.G., and Simon, J.A. (1974). Motor and Leisure Behavior Research Laboratory. University of Illinois, Urbana (unpublished).

Schmidt, R.A. (1972). *Psychonom. Sci.* **27**, 83–85.

Schmidt, R.A., and Russell, D.G. (1972). *J. Exp. Psychol.* **96**, 315–320.

Shields, K.W.D. (1970). Master's Thesis, University of British Columbia (unpublished).

Skoglund, S. (1956). *Acta Physiol. Scand.* **36**, Suppl. 126.

Smith, J.L. (1969). *In* "New Perspectives of Man in Action" (R.C. Brown and B.J. Cratty, eds.), pp. 31–50. Prentice-Hall, Englewood Cliffs, New Jersey.

Stelmach, G.E. (1969). *J. Exp. Psychol.* **81**, 532–536.

Stelmach, G.E. (1970). *J. Mot. Behav.* **2**, 183–194.

Stelmach, G.E. (1974). *In* "Exercise and Sport Sciences Review" (J.H. Wilmore, ed.), Vol. 2, pp. 1–31. Academic Press, New York.

Stelmach, G.E., and Wilson, M. (1970). *J. Exp. Psychol.* **85**, 425–430.

Sussman, H.M. (1972). *Psychol. Bull.* **77**, 262–272.

Taub, D., and Berman, A.J. (1968). *In* "The Neuropsychology of Spatially Oriented Behavior" (S.J. Freedman, ed.), pp. 173–192. Dorsey, Homewood, Illinois.

von Holst, E. (1954). *Brit. J. Anim. Behav.* **2**, 89–94.

Washburn, M.F. (1916). "Movement and Mental Imagery." Houghton, Boston, Massachusetts.

Welford, A.T. (1960). *Ergonomics* **3**, 189–230.

Wickelgren, W.A. (1969). *Psychol. Rev.* **76**, 1–15.

Williams, H.L., Beaver, S.W., Spence, M.T., and Rundell, O.R. (1969). *J. Exp. Psychol.* **80**, 530–536.

Wilson, D.M. (1961). *J. Exp. Psychol.* **38**, 471–485.

Wilson, D.M. (1964). *In* "Neural Theory and Modelling" (R.F. Reiss, ed.), pp. 331–345. Stanford Univ. Press, Stanford, California.

Wood, H. (1969). *J. Exp. Psychol.* **70**, 480–485.

Woodworth, R.S. (1899). *Psychol. Rev.* **3**, Mon. Suppl., No. 3.

Issues for a Closed-Loop
Theory of Motor Learning

Jack A. Adams

I. Introduction

In 1971 I published a paper on a closed-loop theory of human motor learning (Adams, 1971). The ideas of the paper were motivated by shortcomings in open-loop conceptions of motor learning that had dominated the field since its beginning, and by the weaknesses in extant closed-loop descriptions of motor behavior that were little more than interesting analogies drawn from servo theory in engineering. These engineering models were uninteresting to learning psychologists because they had strict assumptions which behavior could not abide, they did not contain learning variables, and they were not rooted in empirical findings for motor behavior (Adams, 1961). I sought to avoid the pitfalls of earlier closed-loop theorists by operationally defining the constructs of my theory so that it could be empirically tested, by including variables which are known to influence motor learning, and by securing the theory in empirical data. It is my conviction that the formulation of good theory is grounded in empirical data. Theory not fixed in data can be a fanciful dream that will have little chance of saying anything about the real world, and it can have an apparent scientific pertinence that is attractive to the unwary.

Today there are ideas abroad in the realm of motor behavior which suggest that it is time to change and enlarge motor theory. This trend is a natural progression in science and is to be encouraged, but some of the recommendations for change are ideas which are thin for want of empirical support and which are poor candidates for theory, at least by the canons of theorizing which guide me. The recommendations most frequently heard are to incorporate the concepts of motor program and schema into theory. After summarizing my closed-loop theory of motor learning as a background for the discussion, I will take a critical look at these scientific concepts and document their ineligibility for formal theory status at this time.

II. Review of Adams' Closed-Loop Theory of Motor Learning

The starting points for my closed-loop theory of motor learning were doubts that I had raised about open-loop conceptions of behavior (Adams, 1967, 1968), and some closed-loop theorizing which I had attempted for paired-associate learning (Adams and Bray, 1970). A stimulus for my theorizing was a discontent with the S-R reinforcement view of learning.

The S-R reinforcement position of learning is one of empirical reinforcement. Any event that follows a response, is correlated with its occurrence, and produces an increment in the probability of occurrence for the response class, is considered a reinforcer. The food pellet which the rat receives when he presses the bar in a Skinner box is a reinforcer because it increases the chances that he will press it again, and the experimenter saying "Right" when the subject draws a 3-in. line is a reinforcer because it increases the probability that he will draw it again. There is no theory of reinforcement that explains the action of these diverse reinforcer events with a common principle. This lack of conceptual elegance does not destroy the scientific usefulness of empirical reinforcement because a great deal of prediction and control of behavior can be exerted with the various reinforcing events that are known to affect behavior.

In motor learning, and often in verbal learning, we call an empirical reinforcing event "knowledge of results," and there is reason to believe that the empirical reinforcement position is wanting and that we can begin to go beyond surface correlations and specify underlying processes. The literature suggests three of these processes:

1. An empirical reinforcement interpretation of knowledge of results says that information about the correctness of the response will lead to an increase in occurrence of the response. Elwell and Grindley (1938) observed that a subject in a motor learning experiment does not repeat a response like a pigeon repeating a key-pecking response for grain reward. Rather, the subject attempts to vary responses and correct error, not repeat responses.

2. Motor behavior is guided by covert verbal behavior in the early stages of learning. Subjects accompany the learning process with hidden verbal activity, where they form hypotheses and plans about the next movement on the basis of the knowledge of results which they have just received. Perhaps from the days when motor behavior was studied by physiologists as a "spinal" activity, there have been those who have identified motor behavior with the lower senses and remote from the upper reaches of the mind. Actually, motor behavior is draped with more cognitive activity than most are willing to admit. The acknowledgment of a role for verbal factors in motor learning does not mean that motor behavior is always under verbal control, however. As William James (1890a,b) said a long time ago, motor sequences are under verbal control at the outset of learning but eventually become "automatic," or nonverbal, as the learning becomes advanced.

3. The error in a motor movement is known by the subject. We have self-knowledge of the adequacy of our movements, and we regulate them on the basis of it.

I believe that we can be carried beyond an empirical reinforcement view of motor learning by incorporating these three processes in a closed-loop theory of motor learning. In my 1971 paper, I distinguished between open-loop and closed-loop systems in the following way:

> An *open-loop* system has no feedback or mechanisms for error regulation. The input events for a system exert their influence, the system effects its transformation on the input, and the system has an output. A poorly operating open-loop system (error) is because of characteristics of the input and/or transformations imposed by the system. A traffic light with fixed timing snarls traffic when the load is heavy and impedes the flow when traffic is light. The system has no compensatory capability.
>
> A *closed-loop* system has feedback, error detection, and error correction as key elements. There is a reference that specifies the desired value for the system, and the output of the system is fed back and compared to the reference for error detection and, if necessary, corrected. The automatic home furnace is a common example. The thermostat setting is the desired value, and the heat output of the furnace is fed back and compared against this reference. If there is a discrepancy the furnace cuts in or out until the error is zero. A closed-loop system is self-regulating by compensating for deviations from the reference [p. 116].

The empirical reinforcement conception of motor learning is open-loop. The response outcome for the system is primarily determined by system changes which reinforcement has made, which has often been conceptualized as habit. By contrast, a closed-loop system has a reference mechanism that specifies the correct response required of the system, feedback which informs of the response which the system has made, a comparison of feedback with the reference mechanism for a determination of error, and a correction of error. An open-loop system treats errors incidentally as evidence of system incompetence because the focus is on occurrences of the correct response, but errors and their processing lie at the center of a closed-loop system.

The trick for devising a closed-loop theory of motor learning is to specify how the mechanisms of a closed-loop system link to learning variables. How is the reference mechanism learned so the subject comes to know when he is performing correctly? What are the sources of feedback and how do they work? What role does knowledge of results play?

A. Knowledge of Results

An interpretation of knowledge of results can be in direct empirical terms, where it is an event whose occurrence affects response probability, but the empirical reinforcement view is insensitive to the fertile workings of the human mind and the operations that it performs on knowledge of results in behalf of the next try at the motor response. One does not have to introspect very hard to know that motor learning can be a problem-solving situation, where the verbal human takes the knowledge of results that he receives and uses his language capabilities to form strategies and hypotheses about how to solve the motor problem that is confronting him. Knowledge of results is information, and how the subject will transform and use it will depend on the type and accuracy of knowledge of results and on the kind of motor task.

B. The Reference Mechanism

A movement must be started, and it must have direction and extent. The starting of the movement is a separate problem, and it will be dealt with in the next section. This section deals with the continuous regulation of the movement once it has started.

The learning of a movement in closed-loop theory requires the acquisition of a reference mechanism which is the basis of the subject knowing the correctness of a response insofar as he has learned it. In addition, the subject needs knowledge of results to inform him about the correctness of the last movement, and response-produced feedback stimuli to inform about the progress of the current movement. The reference mechanism is called the perceptual trace in my theory. At the start of a trial the perceptual trace is aroused in anticipation of feedback from the forthcoming movement, and as the movement proceeds the feedback is compared with it and the appropriateness of the movement is assessed. If the perceptual trace and the feedback match the error signal is zero, and the subject proceeds confidently with the movement. But if the match is absent and there is error, the subject has reduced confidence in the correctness of the movement and moves to eliminate the error. The process is one of continuous error nulling throughout the course of the movement.

The strength of the perceptual trace is a positive function of experience with the various sources of feedback in the situation. Motor movements will have proprioceptive feedback associated with them, and often there is visual feedback as well as auditory and tactual feedback. The perceptual trace is a motor image (not necessarily a conscious one), and the comparison of feedback stimuli with it is an act of recognition, just as the image of a picture from visual experience is the basis for recognizing the picture when it is presented again. The perceptual trace is conveniently referred to as a single state, but actually it is considered to be a distribution of traces resulting from the responses of all of the learning trials. The movement on each trial lays down a trace.

One might stop in this point in the theorizing because the essentials of a closed-loop system have been achieved, but the theory would be pale stuff for learning because it would not have tied the important learning variable of knowledge of results to the perceptual trace and feedback stimuli. A simple error-nulling system will not do because in the beginning the perceptual trace is ill-defined and if the subject adjusted his behavior with respect to it he would be repeating his own errors, which is failure to learn. Instead of repeating his past responses, he must vary his behavior and make his next response different from the last one. The perceptual trace is stored information about past movements that have been made, and knowledge of results is information about the adequacy of the last movement that was made, and the subject uses the two in relation to one another to make the next move better than the last one. The result over trials is the gradual improvement which we call learning. Because knowledge of results and the verbal behavior based on it has a strong role at this stage, it is called the Verbal-Motor Stage. As learning progresses, and the subject has been making little or no error for some time, the perceptual trace becomes a solid reference for the correct response and the subject can now respond with respect to the perceptual trace alone by comparing feedback with it and nulling the perceived error. Knowledge of results is no longer needed. This is called the Motor Stage.

C. The Starting of the Movement

Elsewhere (Adams, 1971, pp. 125–126) I have discussed the logical and empirical reasons for a separate theoretical state, distinct from the perceptual trace, whose function is the initiation and selection of movement. I call this agent the memory trace. Once a movement has started the perceptual trace and feedback regulate it, but it takes the memory trace to start it in the first place.

III. The Motor Program

My closed-loop theory relies fundamentally on response-produced, peripheral feedback stimuli and the perceptual trace, which is the reference of correctness, for the regulation of movement. This structure gives the theory its closed-loop quality, and it has historical continuity with closed-loop theory from engineering which uses peripheral feedback as a source of information about the system's response.

The challenge to a closed-loop view of motor behavior is an open-loop version that is based on the motor program The motor program has a centrally stored plan for the movement sequence, and the plan controls the movement during its course. The implication is that feedback is unnecessary for the regulation of movement, although it has been suggested that feedback is used intermittently to report on the movement's progress and to adjust the ongoing motor program (Keele, 1973, Chapter 6; MacNeilage, 1970). Being central, the motor program is a challenge to revise my closed-loop theory of motor learning because my theory turns strongly on peripheral feedback for movement regulation. It pays, therefore, to examine the empirical foundations of the motor program concept.

At the outset I must point out that a very limited idea of a motor program is necessary for any theory of movement because a movement must be started and feedback does not occur until a fraction of a second later. My concept of memory trace performs the movement initiation function, so in this restricted sense I am an advocate of the motor program. The standard view of the motor program, which comes down to us in the history of motor learning, is not concerned with movement initiation but with extended movement sequences like moving the arm, swinging a bat and hitting a ball, or running down a maze. That there is a central agent which runs off long motor sequences without feedback is the issue.

A. Deafferentation

1. K.S. Lashley, The Founder of the Motor
   Program Hypothesis

The strongest platform for the motor program is deafferentation, where the nerve fibers from the muscles and joints to the motor centers of the brain are cut and the behavioral competence of the organism is observed. That some competence is found in the absence of proprioceptive feedback is taken as support for the central control of movement and a downgrading of feedback.

Lashley (1917) invented the motor program hypothesis during a clinical study of a patient who had gunshot injury to the spinal cord, which is accidental deafferentation. Lashley found that the blindfolded patient never made a mistake in the direction of a voluntary movement, and accuracy in the extent of movement compared favorably with a control subject. From that time on Lashley was a centralist who denied the role of feedback in movement regulation, and he led a crusade against feedback with experiment and argument for the rest of his life. The campaign began with this statement in the 1917 paper:

> We may conclude that the anesthetic subject's control of his movements is not significantly less accurate than that of the normal individual, and it is not clear that for the simple movement studied the afferent impulses from the moving limb contributed anything to the accuracy of movement in the normal subject. The chief mechanism for the control of movement is located in some other body segment than that of the moving organ [p. 185].

The clinical work was only a clue, but Lashley saw it and moved it into the laboratory where he subjected his feedback ideas to experimental attack. Lashley and McCarthy (1926) used rats and insulted the cerebellum with lesions and found that the earlier learning of a complex maze was retained rather well. Lashley and Ball (1929) denied proprioceptive feedback by cutting the spinal afferent paths and they also found good retention of maze performance. Here again Lashley spoke for a central organization of motor activity.

Lashley was not without his critics. W.S. Hunter was a prominent experimental psychologist on the American scene for a long time and his analysis of Lashley's position cut it with surgical neatness. Hunter (1930) said that maze running is behaviorally complex, involving virtually all of the senses, and to deny the animals only one sense ally should not impair performance very much. Learning can make some of the other senses informative too, and they remain influential when proprioceptive feedback is denied. Feedback was still guiding behavior and so the concept of the motor program was unjustified, Hunter contended. Pavlov (1932) also sliced at Lashley's position. He made arguments similar to Hunter's, and at one point (Pavlov, 1932, p. 114) dismissed Lashley's programming notion as a "bodiless reaction." In turn, Lashley (1931) defended himself, but he had to admit that the motor program was a concept unfulfilled:

> The notion of central processes controlling sequences of behavior was little more than a denial of the adequacy of the motor-chain theory [feedback from one movement segment determines the next, J.A.A.] as an explanation of maze running or of thinking and a suggestion that we can profitably study the central-nervous coordinating process. As an explanatory process it is empty, but it may perhaps be filled by continued research [p. 18].

Hunter, Pavlov, and other critics of Lashley (e.g., Honzik, 1936) were correct in their analyses, of course, but this did not deter Lashley. In his best-known paper (Lashley, 1951), Lashley expressed the program idea again, and the empirical foundations were no stronger than they were twenty years before. The motor program might have been the right idea for the wrong reasons, because later investigators tried different research approaches to it and some claimed support for it. As we shall see in sections that follow, the later studies are not without their difficulties either.

2. Recent Deafferentation Studies

Taub and his associates have been the most persistent pursuers of deafferentation in recent times (Knapp et al., 1963; Taub et al., 1965; Taub and Berman, 1963, 1968; Cohn et al., 1972). Theirs is an attempt to correct some of the difficulties with earlier work, and they interpret their data in favor of the motor program. Advocates of the motor program frequently cite the Taub findings as positive evidence, but there is reason for the enthusiasm to be restrained.

Lashley had the problem that nonproprioceptive sources of feedback could come to guide the response through learning, and Taub and his colleagues have the same problem. Consider the experiment by Knapp et al. (1963). They used monkeys and sought to eliminate visual feedback by strapping an animal in a chair with an opaque collar during avoidance conditioning trials. The conditioned response was forelimb flexion, and the opaque collar obscured vision of it, but not vision of the surrounding room. Correlated movement of the head or eyes could have given visual feedback that would come to be informative about movement progress over learning trials; there is no reason to believe that only visual feedback of the responding limb is informative about the course of movement. Or consider the conditioned stimulus as a source of auditory feedback. The conditioned stimulus was a buzzer which came on for 7 sec and the unconditioned stimulus, an electric shock, came on for the last 3.5 sec. If the animal made the conditioned response the buzzer terminated, which was informative feedback about the movement. One of their findings was that deafferented animals were unable to use the deafferented limbs in a free situation but readily used them to avoid shock in the conditioning situation. The most likely reason seems to be that the conditioning trials created reliable sources of feedback information about movement that were lacking in the free situation.

In subsequent experiments (Taub and Berman, 1963; Taub et al., 1965), feedback from the conditioned stimulus was eliminated by using trace conditioning where the conditioned stimulus is off by the time the unconditioned stimulus and the response occurs, but the same lack of visual control persisted. That visual feedback can provide guidance for deafferented limbs has been found in several studies. Ataxia is greatly accentuated in blindfolded deafferented animals and can be absent without it (Twitchell, 1954; Bossom and Ammaya, 1968; Knapp et al., 1963). Pavlov (1932, p. 188) observed that ataxic subjects with tabes dorsalis can stand on one leg when the eyes are open but fall when the eyes are shut. Leont'ev and Zaporozhets (1960, Chapter 1) studied war veterans who had restricted movements because of battle injuries. Subjects with restricted movement of the shoulder joint were instructed to close their eyes and raise the damaged arm as high as possible. Then they were asked to repeat the act with eyes open. The second movement was $7°$ higher than the first.

If these difficulties are not enough, Bossom and Ammaya (1968) criticize the surgical techniques which Taub and his colleagues use, and suggest the possibility that some dorsal root fibers might have remained intact. If so, this is a serious criticism because the existence of only a few fibers is sufficient for coordinated behavior after recovery from surgery (Bossom and Ammaya, 1968; Mott and Sherrington, 1895; Twitchell, 1954). Recently a paper from Taub's laboratory (Cohn et al., 1972) discussed the difficulties with the surgical procedures in deafferentation. As an added check on the completeness of the deafferentation, they tested to see if motor movement could produce evoked potentials at the cortex. None were found, and they asserted confidence in their current surgical methods.

So, like Lashley, all that Taub and his colleagues have shown is that skilled responding is possible without proprioceptive feedback, not that the motor program is a valid concept. There can be no test of the motor program hypothesis in the absence of controls on the other sources of feedback that can come to be endowed with informative properties for movement through learning. Even the autonomic nervous system can provide cues for movement, and learning psychologists have used this possibility in their theorizing. For example, Mowrer (1947) had fear stimuli as the cues for motor avoidance responses in his two-factor theory of emotional learning. In the literature domain that is particularly pertinent to our inquiry here, Mott and Sherrington (1895), Twitchell (1954), and Bossom and Ammaya (1968) found that a deafferented animal can have his coordination restored when he is emotionally aroused, suggesting a role for emotional stimuli in the maintenance of manipulative and ambulatory movements. Perhaps the fundamental observation is not that we can move without proprioception but that learning can make any source of feedback informative for movement.

B. The Motor Program as a Determiner
of Certain Insect Behaviors

It is common for advocates of the motor program to cite research on insect behavior as a strong line of positive evidence for the program idea, and it is justified. Experimental biologists have amassed evidence for feedback-free behavior (Hinde, 1969a,b; Evarts et al., 1971, Chapter 2), and this is the kind of behavior that supports the program concept. The best-known work is by Wilson (1964, 1965) on the wingbeat of the locust. The sexual behavior of the mantis and the cockroach is held to be programmed (Roeder et al., 1960). Insect walking behavior is under a degree of programmed control (Pearson, 1972;

Pearson and Iles, 1973; Wilson, 1966). That the concept of the motor program is applicable to the insect domain is important to know because it means that the idea has some validity, but to leap from genetically determined behavior in insects to learned behavior in animals, including man, is a jump that is too large for many scientific temperaments. That biological evolution can genetically determine behavioral sequences is grounded empirically and believed by us all, but the issue is learning, the ultimate in adaptability, not restricted programmed sequences which genetics has endowed.

C. Proprioception and the Control of Fast Movement

Always, defenders of the motor program move Lashley's (1951) example of the pianist to center stage. The anecdote has it that a pianist's fingers can move at the rate of 16/sec, and this is too fast for closed-loop proprioceptive feedback control of movement. Lashley's anecdote continues to be a compelling example for some, despite modern physiological research on proprioception and the fact that no one has ever bothered to measure the speed of a pianist's fingers. The serial ordering of speech is an instructive example on the control of fast movements. Is speech a series of open-loop commands, or is tactual and proprioceptive feedback control sufficiently swift to do the regulatory job?

MacNeilage (1970) admits to a possible role of the closed-loop control of speech, but mainly he defends open-loop programmed control where the target end points are specified and the muscles can take various routes to them. Implicit throughout his paper is the sentiment that proprioceptive feedback is not fast enough to control the speech apparatus. Most psychologists, in conducting this argument, cite Chernikoff and Taylor's (1952) finding that kinesthetic reaction time is 119 msec. It is true that if the motor stimulation-brain-motor response loop ordinarily took this long to operate it would be difficult to argue for closed-loop control. However, as we shall see in this section, modern work on the physiology of proprioception provides lines of evidence which show that proprioceptive feedback can be much faster than the work of Chernikoff and Taylor implies, and so a closed-loop interpretation is becoming more plausible than ever before. Sussman (1972), in a reply to MacNeilage (1970), has speech as his battlefield and marshals his physiological evidence and his closed-loop forces very effectively. His arguments are secured in the physiological research of Bowman (1968) and Bowman and Combs (1968, 1969a,b) on muscle spindles in the monkey's tongue. The tongue is a remarkably skilled organ when we stop to think about it. Its intricate positioning and timing in the oral cavity is a prime factor in that complex learned activity which we call intelligible speech, and the tongue's skills may be a good focus for some of these issues that concern us.

Muscle spindles are absent in the tongue of lower animals like the cat, but not so for primates. The monkey and the human tongue have their intrinsic and extrinsic muscles richly laced with spindles (Bowman, 1968), and they are arranged in transverse, vertical, and longitudinal dimensions to communicate the position of the tongue in three-dimensional space (Bowman and Combs, 1968). Ten different response patterns of the stretch sensitive units of the hypoglossal nerve were identified. Different amounts of stretch gave different amounts of impulse frequencies, and many of the stretch sensitive units gave velocity responses during the dynamic phase of the stretch. Moreover, the lingual nerve responded to stretch in any direction and with an acceleration in their discharge frequency. The adequate stimulus for the lingual nerve was distortion of the tongue's surface. Bowman and Combs (1968) see the sensors of the tongue as the structural substrate for a "highly discriminative feedback system [p. 117]." Sussmann (1972), in his comment on these findings, said:

> The finding by Bowman and Combs substantiates the view that there is a vast potential existing within the oral cavity for a detailed, one-to-one mapping of the oral area onto corresponding cortical areas. Hence, the two neural systems (hypoglossal and lingual) can provide an extensive repertoire of information to the higher control centers to bring about closed-loop control of target attainment during the articulatory gestures of speech [p. 269].

A subsequent study by Bowman and Combs (1969a) is a reply to the argument that there is insufficient time for the brain to be informed about movement. Stimulation of the monkey's hypoglossal nerve produced cortical potentials with a latency of 4–5 msec. Other studies have shown an equally fast response. Bowman and Combs (1969b) stimulated the deep radial nerve of the monkey's elbow and obtained a response in the cerebellum in 4 msec.

Fuchs and Kornhuber (1969) found that stretch of the extraocular muscle of the cat produced a response in the cerebellum in 4 msec and a response in the brain stem in 3–4 msec. Citing evidence by Cohen et al. (1965) that the time from the cerebellum back to the eye muscle takes 5.5 msec, Fuchs and Kornhuber estimate the time for the complete trip from muscle receptor to brain back to eye muscles to be 10 msec. Evarts (1973) studied the motor input of a learned hand movement, where a monkey was taught to move a handle back to a correct position after it had been mechanically displaced. Cortical and EMG responses were recorded. The time from the motor stimulus to a cortical response was 10 msec. EMG response to the motor stimulus (cortically mediated) was only 30–40 msec. In a similar fashion, Sears and Davis (1968) used a human subject and made EMG recordings in the respiratory muscles to a change in pressure load on the lungs. They obtained a latency of the EMG response in the 50–60 msec range. Proponents of the motor program have always assumed that the motor system does not have the neural speed for the closed-loop regulation of movement, but these recent physiological research findings suggest otherwise. Lashley's pianist may be a closed-loop system after all.

D. The Motor Program, Feedback, and Learning

Motor program advocates are concerned with memory but they are not much interested in the learning operations that store the movement sequence in memory in the first place, so they fail to specify how the program is acquired. Is feedback irrelevant throughout the learning of a program? Or does feedback only play a role early in learning, with the program being a developing independence of feedback as learning progresses? An experiment by Adams et al. (1972) was designed to test these possibilities. Linear positioning was the task that they used, and it was learned under either augmented feedback or minimal feedback. With augmented feedback there was full vision, the subject could hear the slide which he manipulated move along its track, and he had spring tension on the slide to give heightened proprioceptive feedback. Minimal feedback was none of these. After low or high amount of practice with knowledge of results, the knowledge of results was withdrawn and the feedback either remained the same or was switched, depending upon the experimental condition. If the motor program is independent of feedback throughout its learning then feedback change should make no difference whether the amount of learning was low or high. But if the learning of a program is gradual liberation from feedback, then feedback change should produce a performance difference at the low level of learning but not the high level. Neither of these things happened. Feedback change made a big difference for both levels of learning. Moreover, the difference was the greatest for the high level of learning, which is contrary to the possibility that a motor program develops with practice. The authors interpret their data in support of my closed-loop theory of motor learning which has a role for feedback throughout all stages of learning.

E. Error Detection and Correction

My closed-loop theory of motor learning uses a comparison of the perceptual trace and peripheral feedback for the determination of error. We know that feedback is fundamental for motor sequences (e.g., Adams, 1968) but an issue for closed-loop theory is more specific than that: Does feedback play a role in error detection and correction? An experiment by Adams and Goetz (1973) took deliberate aim at this question. They found that the accuracy of error detection and correction was positively related to amount of feedback and amount of practice, as my theory contends.

When one's theoretical stance is the motor program, where feedback is played down, there is the problem of accounting for error detection. How is it done? MacNeilage (1970) and Keele (1973, Chapter 6) use the motor program to generate the movement but with response-produced feedback stimuli entering intermittently, reporting on movement error and modifying the program if necessary. This is a compromise hypothesis which seems very difficult to test. It is insufficient to show that either the motor program or feedback are governing agents for movement (the issue which is in the center of our scientific eye at the moment). Rather, it must be shown that both the motor program and feedback are operating and, also, the circumstances of their interaction must be demonstrated.

Corollary Discharge

Defenders of the motor program are looking with increasing fondness at corollary discharge to assume a burden in error determination. Corollary discharge is central feedforward stimuli, in contrast to feedback stimuli. Supposedly, the motor program discharges stimuli about the movement-to-be to sensory centers of the brain where there is a comparison with an image representation of the desired movement and error is determined. An idea like this seems required for a motor program approach because if feedback stimuli are unimportant then error assessment must come from other sources, presumably central ones.

The term "corollary discharge" was invented by Sperry (1950) in his research on the visual behavior of fish. He contended that the advent of an eye movement was accompanied by "an anticipatory adjustment in the visual centers specific for each movement with regard to its direction and speed [p. 488]." This idea has been used to explain the old puzzle in visual perception about how we distinguish movement in the world from voluntary movement of the head and eyes. Since both result in movement of visual stimuli on the retina, how do we know one from the other? The answer that is commonly given is that corollary discharge informs the visual centers of the brain that the movement about to be perceived is self-generated, and so the world seems stable in the face of a changing visual scene. The world moves when changing visual stimuli are unaccompanied by corollary discharge. Corollary discharge has been discussed and used by various writers (e.g., Evarts et al., 1971; Konorski, 1962; Taub and Berman, 1968; Teuber, 1964). The empirical validity of a central, anticipatory sensory discharge that is unrelated to external stimuli is established for lower animals (e.g., Johnstone and Mark, 1969, 1971).

The issue for corollary discharge is not whether it exists or not but how much information it carries. For a motor program notion to work the situation must arouse an image representation (or what I call the perceptual trace) in anticipation of the response-to-be, and the motor program must then transmit the corollary discharge which contains all of the information about the forthcoming movement for a comparison with the image for a determination of error. This means that all of the characteristics of the movement must be coded in the corollary discharge, but there is no evidence that this is so. The empirical data show that there is a signal to a sensory center of the brain but no one knows how much information it carries. Perhaps it is only a simple signal of the movement, with no information about movement features whatsoever. Certainly the argument that is made about the explanatory value of corollary discharge for eye movements and visual perception can be sustained with a simple corollary discharge signal. For a stable visual world, the brain need only know that the eye is about to move, not the speed, direction, and terminal position of the move. In my theory, corollary discharge could be the anticipatory signal that galvanizes the perceptual trace to action and readies it for the feedback that will arrive when the movement is begun.

The use of corollary discharge as a sister concept of the motor program is in the weak tradition of physiological explanations of behavior because there has been no bridging of the interface between physiological and behavioral data. The research on deafferentation is on sounder ground because physiological indices of feedback, or its absence, are directly related to behavior in the same experiments. If experiments on deafferentation and motor behavior were done in the same way as the experiments on corollary discharge and motor behavior, there would be studies that would cut afferent fibers and show their failure to transmit proprioceptive stimuli, and there would be other studies that would show motor behavior related to proprioceptive stimuli, but there would be no experiments that related deafferentation and motor behavior in the same experiment. We have yet to show a direct relationship between corollary discharge and motor competence.

IV. Schema

My closed-loop theory of motor learning has each movement separately generated and its stimulus consequences separately stored. The advocates of schema for motor behavior contend, as a counterproposal, that what really happens is that a general plan for a class of movements develops which the performer flexibly uses to respond to the momentary demands of the situation. There are many response routes to the same goal, and a schema allow any one of them to be chosen. This generalized plan for a class of movements will be called the recall schema, and it is closely analogous to concept behavior. To know a concept is to be able to recognize an instance of a stimulus class even though it has never been experienced before. To have the concept "three" is to know three objects even though a particular aggregation of three objects has never been encountered before (e.g., three Martian maidens). The recall schema, it is contended, will allow you to make a movement of a class even though you have never made that particular movement before.

Schema has been used so often to explain findings in visual recognition that one might think that it was devised for that purpose, but not so. The schema was first used by the British neurosurgeon Henry Head to explain aspects of motor behavior. Head's interest in motor behavior came out of his neurological studies of the injured of World War I (Head, 1920a,b), but his research on aphasia is also classic (Head, 1926a,b), and Frederic C. Bartlett collaborated with him on it. Bartlett, being a psychologist, brought the schema into psychology to explain verbal recall primarily, and it is Bartlett's version (1932) which most psychologists know. The schema also is used to explain form recognition (e.g., Attneave, 1957) and motor recall (Bartlett, 1932; Bernstein, 1967; Bruner, 1970; MacNeilage, 1970; Pew, 1970, 1974; Schmidt, 1975). In order to understand schema, and to assess its credibility for modern theory of motor behavior, it is instructive to trace the convolutions of the schema concept from its beginning with Head. The different meanings of schema have not always been appreciated.

A. Three Conceptions of Schema

1. Head's Conception of the Schema

That motor images are influential in the evaluation of movement was an idea prevalent in the early part of this century, and Head rejected it. Allow a patient with sensory damage to his arm to see its position, and then have him close his eyes. Change the position of the arm with the eyes remaining closed and ask the patient about the location of his arm. He will say that his arm is in its original position, not the changed position, and Head said that this is because he has a visual image of the original position of the arm but no motor image to inform him of the move and the second position. A conscious motor image, then, cannot be the basis of movement recognition, said Head. Theorizing anew, Head (1920b, pp. 604–608) defined a spatiotemporal model of movement which is derived from experience and which is the internal standard for the recognition of movement. Head (1920b) wrote:

> For this combined standard, against which all subsequent changes of posture are measured before they enter consciousness, we propose the word "schema." By means of perpetual alterations in position we are always building up a postural model of ourselves which constantly changes. Every new posture of movement is recorded on this plastic schema, and the activity of the cortex brings every fresh group of sensations evoked by altered posture into relation with it. Immediate postural recognition follows as soon as the relation is complete [p. 605].

Schema for Head is the internal reference for response recognition. It resembles my concept of perceptual trace (or vice versa).

2. Bartlett's Conception of the Schema

Bartlett's use of the schema (1932, Chapter 10) has two thrusts. One was accounting for his data on the recall of prose, and the other was accounting for the motor behavior in popular British sports. Bartlett related these disparate topics with the schema.

Bartlett's work on verbal recall had his subjects learn a brief story and then recall it repeatedly after various retention intervals. Bartlett found that the core of the story's idea usually would be retained and, according to Bartlett, would be used to reconstruct the details of the story, some of them correct and some of them not. Bartlett's use of the schema as the central idea that is stored, and from which the protocol at recall is constructed, not only accounts for Bartlett's empirical findings but was, at the same time, a rejection of an account of memory where each response element at recall is based on a separate memory trace. The stored agent is a generalized schema, according to Bartlett, not a set of separate memory traces, and the schema gives a measure of creativity in responding because responses can occur which have never been made before.

Bartlett reasoned the same about motor movement. The execution of movement is not the activation of a passive set of memory traces. Rather, the movement which occurs is never exactly old or completely new but is "manufactured" out of the postural and situational schemata that prevail. Skill in a complex game like tennis does not come from practice and storage of the large number of moves that comprise proficiency, but rather is the development of a much smaller number of schemata that allow the required movements to be created to meet the demands of the situation.

For our purposes here, the important thing to notice about Bartlett's position is that he gave Head's concept of the schema a new function. Head used schema as the internal model for response recognition, but Bartlett used it for the generation of responses—the schema became the basis of recall.

3. Attneave's Conception of the Schema

Attneave (1957) is responsible for bringing the concept of schema to the realm of stimulus (form, pattern) recognition. A classical view of pattern recognition is template matching where experience with the stimulus stores a representation of the stimulus pattern in memory, which has often been called an image. At the recognition test the stimulus is presented again, and if the image is aroused the subject will say that he recognizes it. A variation of template matching is feature matching, where only key features of the stimulus are stored. Another possibility is that the proper kind of experience with members of a defined class of stimuli can result in the storage of a more general representation of the pattern, or an abstraction of the pattern. The abstraction subsumes particular stimulus instances, in the same fashion that a concept subsumes particular instances, and it gives the power to recognize all of them. Given the abstract pattern, a subject can recognize instances of a pattern that have never been experienced before. Attneave gave empirical credibility to this idea, and he called the stored abstraction of a class of forms a schema.

Head used schema as an explanatory mechanism for response recognition, and Bartlett used it for recall, but Attneave had schema as the mechanism for stimulus recognition.

B. The Empirical Validity of Schema

Three uses of schema have been identified, and users of schema have not always been meticulous in specifying their meaning of schema and distinguishing it from other meanings. Notwithstanding, the human has undeniable powers of abstraction, and schema seems to have been the label that various analysts have used for conceptlike behavior when they thought they had identified it. To what extent have these analysts produced acceptable empirical evidence for the three kinds of schema that have stepped forward in the past fifty years or so? If theory must have guidance from substantive empirical data to embrace a concept, to what extent are these three kinds of schema ready for their theoretical debut?

1. Stimulus Recognition Schema

This is the schema that has the strongest support of all. Research on this version of the schema has accelerated in recent years and a satisfying amount of empirical support has developed for it (e.g., Attneave, 1957; Charness and Bregmen, 1973; Peterson *et al.*, 1973; Posner *et al.*, 1967; Posner and Keele, 1968; Posner, 1969). The experimental paradigm for developing a schema is experience with the prototype of the stimulus class or with varied instances of the stimulus class. It is not contended that the schema explains all recognition, because it is unlikely that a schema will develop after only one brief exposure to a stimulus, and yet we have power to recognize it. Nevertheless, we have good capability for recognizing all instances of a stimulus class (all triangles, all humans) even though we have directly experienced only a subset of them.

2. Recall Schema

Schema means versatility, and the recall schema is response versatility where the subject has the option of various response routes to the goal. Bartlett's skilled tennis player has, say, the goal of placing the ball in the far left corner, and he can elect various behavioral routes to fulfill this plan. The performer is not stimulus-response bound, where he must have practiced all of the possible moves that a proficient game requires. Once the schema has been acquired he can make responses that he has never made before.

The discomforting problem with recall schema for skills is that there is no reliable evidence for it. From Bartlett's intuition about skills and his background with Head came the hypothesis of recall schema, but his evidence in behalf of skills was anecdotal accounts of feats on the courts and playing fields. Perceptive analyses of everyday behavior can be the beginning of a worthy scientific hypothesis, but only a beginning. First analyses of this sort hardly qualify as empirical data that can support a theoretical concept. Bartlett's versatile tennis player could have had thousands of hours of practice, as is common among skilled athletes, and instead of recall schema it is just as reasonable to believe that practice has been given to the many moves that make up his impressive game. Couple this practice with some verbal control of motor behavior (Adams, 1971), and we have an alternative account of versatile skills.

A good starting point for research on motor recall schema would be something like the paradigm that is used to test stimulus recognition schema. The experimental design should be a transfer of training design, and as a minimum it should contain the conditions shown in the following tabulation:

Group	Training	Transfer
Experimental	Training on varied instances of a class of motor responses	All groups transfer to one or more new instances of the motor response class
Control I	Training on a single instance of the class of motor responses	
Control II		

If a recall schema has developed the Experimental Group will perform better than the control groups on the transfer test. Maybe Control Group I will perform better than Control Group II on the transfer test. Adams (1954) and Morrisett and Hovland (1959) found positive transfer under such circumstances in a problem-solving task.

This would seem to be an easy experiment to run, and yet it will not be easy because so many motor responses have accompanying verbal behavior; the recall schema may be no more than a consistent verbal mediator that is guiding the motor response. Suppose the motor response class chosen for study is the drawing of circles. The Experimental Group draws many different kinds of circles in training and all subjects covertly label their motor responses with the same verbal description each time. Assume that the repeated drawing of a single circle by Control Group I leads to less frequent labeling. In the transfer test the subjects of the Experimental Group could say to themselves "He wants me to draw a circle again," and they would proceed to do so. Control Group I subjects label less frequently and perform less well on the test and so the conclusion would be in behalf of a motor recall schema. The conclusion would be inappropriate because it is an experiment on verbal mediation as a determinant of motor behavior, not recall schema.

If a motor recall schema means no more than verbal mediation then we know more about it than we think we do. I am quite sure, however, that motor recall schema is intended to mean a wholly motor agent which might sometimes have verbal accompaniment but which is quite capable of producing motor versatility alone. To get at the fundamental motor core of motor recall schema will be difficult because of the ubiquitousness of verbal behavior. Possible research possibilities are to use motor sequences that defy verbal description, or to use preverbal children or animals. Another difficulty will be the definition of a motor response class. It is one thing to define a class of patterns for stimulus recognition experiments (all triangles, all dwellings), and quite another to define a class of movements whose definition sets it off from other classes of movement.

3. Response Recognition Schema

The recall schema has anecdotal evidence in shaky support of it but the response recognition schema lacks even that. The gist of the response recognition schema is that the subject can develop a capability to recognize and decide about the appropriateness of a class of motor responses, even though some of them have never occurred before. Response recognition is the function which I give to the perceptual trace in my closed-loop theory of motor learning, but I have the sensory consequences of each motor movement stored and entering a distribution of traces, which becomes a primary governing agent for the behavior. My theory would say that a movement outside the distribution of responses that has not been practiced would be poorly recognized as a member of the class, but the concept of response recognition schema would predict otherwise (providing the new response can be defended as a member of the motor response class).

V. General Conclusions

A theory to be scientifically fruitful must receive good guidance from empirical data when it is conceived, as I said in the beginning of this chapter, and I believe that the concepts of motor program and schema are insufficiently supported at this time to be given meaningful definitions in motor theory; they should be held in the wings and regarded as pretheoretical until data justify moving them on to the stage that is theory. So I am temporarily satisfied with the omission of motor program and schema from my closed-loop theory of motor learning, although I am fascinated with the research challenge that they pose.

References

Adams, J.A. (1954). *J. Exp. Psychol.* **48**, 15–18.
Adams, J.A. (1961). *Psychol. Bull.* **58**, 55–79.

Adams, J.A. (1967). "Human Memory." McGraw-Hill, New York.

Adams, J.A. (1968). *Psychol. Bull.* **70**, 486–504.

Adams, J.A. (1971). *J. Mot. Behav.* **3**, 111–149.

Adams, J.A., and Bray, N.W. (1970). *Psychol. Rev.* **77**, 385–405.

Adams, J.A., and Goetz, E.T. (1973). *J. Mot. Behav.* **5**, 217–224.

Adams, J.A., Goetz, E.T., and Marshall, P.H. (1972). *J. Exp. Psychol.* **92**, 391–397.

Attneave, F. (1957). *J. Exp. Psychol.* **54**, 81–88.

Bartlett, F.C. (1932). "Remembering: A Study in Experimental and Social Psychology." Univ. of Cambridge Press, London and New York.

Bernstein, N. (1967). "The Co-ordination and Regulation of Movements." Pergamon, Oxford.

Bossom, J., and Ommaya, A.K. (1968). *Brain* **91**, 161–172.

Bowman, J.P. (1968). *Anat. Rec.* **161**, 483–488.

Bowman, J.P., and Combs, C.M. (1968). *Exp. Neurol.* **21**, 105–119.

Bowman, J.P., and Combs, C.M. (1969a). *Exp. Neurol.* **23**, 291–301.

Bowman, J.P., and Combs, C.M. (1969b). *Exp. Neurol.* **23**, 537–543.

Bruner, J.S. (1970). *In* "Mechanisms of Motor Skill Development" (K. Connolly, ed.), pp. 63–92. Academic Press, New York.

Charness, N., and Bregman, A.S. (1973). *Can. J. Psychol.* **27**, 367–380.

Chernikoff, R., and Taylor, F.V. (1952). *J. Exp. Psychol.* **43**, 1–8.

Cohen, B., Goto, K., Shanzer, S., and Weiss, A.H. (1965). *Exp. Neurol.* **13**, 145–162.

Cohn, R., Jakniunas, A., and Taub, E. (1972). *Science* **178**, 1113–1115.

Elwell, J.L., and Grindley, G.C. (1938). *Brit. J. Psychol.* **29**, 39–54.

Evarts, E.V. (1973). *Science* **179**, 501–503.

Evarts, E.V., Bizzi, E., Burke, R.E., DeLong, M., and Thach, W.T., Jr. (1971). *Neurosci. Res. Program, Bull.* **9**, Whole No. 1.

Fuchs, A.F., and Kornhuber, H.H. (1969). *J. Physiol. (London)* **200**, 713–722.

Head, H. (1920a). "Studies in Neurology," Vol. I. Oxford Univ. Press, London and New York.

Head, H. (1920b). "Studies in Neurology," Vol. II. Oxford Univ. Press, London and New York.

Head, H. (1926a). "Aphasia and Kindred Disorders of Speech," Vol. I. Macmillan, New York.

Head, H. (1926b). "Aphasia and Kindred Disorders of Speech," Vol. II. Macmillan, New York.

Hinde, R.A. (1969a). "Animal Behaviour." McGraw Hill, New York.

Hinde, R.A. (1969b). *Quart. J. Exp. Psychol.* **21**, 105–126.

Honzik, C.H. (1936). *Comp. Psychol. Monogr.* **13**, Whole No. 64.

Hunter, W.S. (1930). *J. Gen. Psychol.* **3**, 455–468.

James, W. (1890a). "Principles of Psychology," Vol. I. Holt, New York.

James, W. (1890b). "Principles of Psychology," Vol. II. Holt, New York.

Johnstone, J.R., and Mark, R.F. (1969). *Comp. Biochem. Physiol.* **30**, 931–939.

Johnstone, J.R., and Mark, R.F. (1971). *J. Exp. Biol.* **54**, 403–414.

Keele, S.W. (1973). "Attention and Human Performance." Goodyear, Pacific Palisades, California.

Knapp, H.D., Taub, E., and Berman, A.J. (1963). *Exp. Neurol.* **7**, 305–315.

Konorski, J. (1962). *Brain* **85**, 277–294.

Lashley, K.S. (1917). *Amer. J. Physiol.* **43**, 169–194.

Lashley, K.S. (1931). *J. Gen. Psychol.* **5**, 3–19.

Lashley, K.S. (1951). *In* "Cerebral Mechanisms in Behavior" (L.A. Jeffress, ed.), pp. 112–136. Wiley, New York.

Lashley, K.S., and Ball, J. (1929). *J. Comp. Psychol.* **9**, 71–106.

Lashley, K.S., and McCarthy, D.A. (1926). *J. Comp. Psychol.* **6**, 423–434.

Leont'ev, A.N., and Zaporozhets, A.V. (1960). "Rehabilitation of Hand Function" (B. Haigh, transl.). Pergamon, Oxford.

MacNeilage, P.F. (1970). *Psychol. Rev.* **77**, 182–196.

Morrisett, L., Jr., and Hovland, C.I. (1959). *J. Exp. Psychol.* **58**, 52–55.

Mott, F.W., and Sherrington, C.S. (1895). *Proc. Roy. Soc.* **57**, 481–488.

Mowrer, O.H. (1947). *Harvard Educ. Rev.* **17**, 102–148.

Pavlov, I.P. (1932). *Psychol. Rev.* **39**, 91–127.

Pearson, K.G. (1972). *J. Exp. Biol.* **56**, 173–192.

Pearson, K.G., and Iles, J.F. (1973). *J. Exp. Biol.* **58**, 725–744.

Peterson, M.J., Meagher, R.B., Jr., Chait, H., and Gillie, S. (1973). *Cog. Psychol.* **4**, 378–398.

Pew, R.W. (1970). *J. Mot. Behav.* **2**, 8–24.

Pew, R.W. (1974). *Hum. Perf. Ctr. Tech. Rep.* No. **48**. Univ. of Michigan, Ann Arbor.

Posner, M.I. (1969). *In* "The Psychology of Learning and Motivation" (G.H. Bower and J.T. Spence, eds.), Vol. 3, pp. 43–100. Academic Press, New York.

Posner, M.I., and Keele, S.W. (1968). *J. Exp. Psychol.* **77**, 353–363.

Posner, M.I., Goldsmith, R., and Welton, K.E., Jr. (1967). *J. Exp. Psychol.* **73**, 28–38.

Roeder, K.D., Tozian, L., and Weiant, E.A. (1960). *J. Insect Physiol.* **4**, 45–62.

Schmidt, R.A. (1975). *Psychol. Rev.* **82**, 225–260.

Sears, T.A., and Davis, J.N. (1968). *Ann. N.Y. Acad. Sci.* **155**, 183–190.

Sperry, R.W. (1950). *J. Comp. Physiol. Psychol.* **43**, 482–489.

Sussmann, H.M. (1972). *Psychol. Bull.* **77**, 262–272.

Taub, E., and Berman, A.J. (1963). *J. Comp. Physiol. Psychol.* **56**, 1012–1016.

Taub, E., and Berman, A.J. (1968). *In* "The Neuropsychology of Spatially Oriented Behavior" (S.J. Freedman, ed.), pp. 173–192. Dorsey, Homewood, Illinois.

Taub, E., Bacon, R.C., and Berman, A.J. (1965). *J. Comp. Physiol. Psychol.* **59**, 275–279.

Teuber, H.-L. (1964). *Acquis. Lang. Mongr. Soc. Res. Child Develop.* **29**, 131–138.

Twitchell, T.E. (1954). *J. Neurophysiol.* **17**, 239–252.

Wilson, D.M. (1964). *In* "Neural Theory and Modeling" (R.F. Reiss, ed.), pp. 331–345. Stanford Univ. Press, Stanford, California.

Wilson, D.M. (1965). *In* "Physiology of the Insect Central Nervous System" (J.E. Treherne and J.W.L. Beament, eds.), pp. 125–140. Academic Press, New York.

Wilson, D.M. (1966). *Annu. Rev. Entemol.* **11**, 103–122.

The Structure
of Motor Programs

Steven W. Keele
Jeffery J. Summers

I. Introduction

A good many motor tasks involve a complex series of movements. The skilled performer often differs from the unskilled performer in such tasks not necessarily in the quickness or precision of individual reactions and movements but in the coordination of the successive movements into a smooth and orderly sequence. When people are unskilled, they make a movement, evaluate the results, make another movement, reevaluate, and so on, and their performance is therefore quite irregular. As they acquire skill, the sequence of movements becomes structured so that it no longer is under direct visual control (Pew, 1966, offers good evidence for such a change). The movements anticipate or coincide with the events in the environment that they are intended to deal with, and they appear coordinated with each other. In other words, the sequence of movements becomes stored in the memory system so that it can be executed without constant correction by reference to the environment. Understanding the mechanism of sequencing clearly is an important element in understanding skilled performance.

This chapter is concerned primarily with the nature of the memory structure that underlies skill. Some evidence will be described that led to a particular theory of sequence representation, namely, motor program theory. Essentially motor program theory posits that the sequencing of a skill is represented centrally and does not require peripheral feedback from prior movements to elicit succeeding movements. This is not to deny, however, the critical role of feedback in skilled performance; consequently, some consideration is also given to its role. After considering some practical applications of the program-feedback model to skill training, a more detailed analysis of the memorial structure will be given. Granted the sequence representation is a motor program, is the movement series stored as event associations, as position associations, as a higher order structure, or perhaps in more than one code? Is timing an integral part of the sequence representation, or is the ordering of events and timing of events separately represented? Questions of this sort will be discussed in the last section of the chapter.

II. The Motor Program Concept

A commonly held, early theory of sequence representation is S-R chaining; it is illustrated in Figure 1 based on Greenwald (1970). Early in practice, as shown in panel A, successive responses are elicited by successive cues in the environment. As a movement is issued a pattern of kinesthetic stimulation unique to the movement flows from the various joint, cutaneous, and stretch receptors in the moving limb. Because the kinesthetic stimulation from one movement occurs just prior to a succeeding movement, the feedback from one movement becomes conditioned to the next (panel B). A basic tenet of classical conditioning is that any stimulation that systematically precedes a response will eventually come to elicit that response. Eventually, therefore, the entire skill can be executed in response to a starting stimulus and in the absence of other external stimuli, because each succeeding response is elicited by the pattern of internal stimuli from the preceding response.

One long-standing argument against S-R chaining as a general theory of movement control is that feedback processing is too slow to account for very rapid sequences of movements such as finger movements in playing the piano

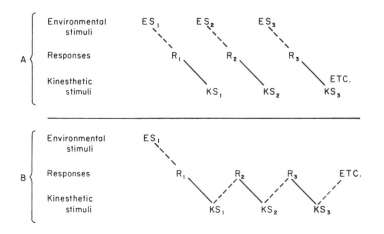

Figure 1 During initial learning of a skill, successive responses are controlled by environmental stimuli (panel A). According to S-R chaining theory, as learning progresses responses become conditioned to the kinesthetic feedback from the preceding response (panel B).

(Glencross, 1975; Lashley, 1951).[1] Many skills involve successive movements at intervals less than 100 msec, and yet the time to react to kinesthetic stimulation was reported to be 100 msec or greater (Glencross, 1975; Keele, 1968). Recently, however, Evarts and Tanji (1974), recording the electrical discharge from the muscles, a procedure more sensitive than those previously used, reported that monkeys can make use of kinesthetic feedback in about 40 or 50 msec. Such a rapid influence of feedback is not simply due to a built-in reflex, and instead involves flexible coupling of feedback to response as would be required for feedback to be useful in skill learning. The monkeys are able to respond by either pushing or pulling in response to the same kinesthetic signal, depending on prior instructions. Built-in reflexes should not be amenable by instruction. Thus, the argument that S-R chaining is impossible because of the time constraints of kinesthetic processing is less persuasive than previously thought.

More convincing evidence contrary to S-R chaining theory comes from studies that surgically eliminated kinesthetic feedback in animals. If the skill can proceed without kinesthesis, then S-R chaining, in which the stimuli are kinesthetic, cannot explain the sequencing. Many studies have in fact shown that movement sequences can be maintained when feedback is removed [Bossom (1974) and Hinde (1969) review several such studies]. Some examples are shown

---

[1] Some people have taken this argument of Lashley's as a general criticism of any associative chaining theory, but it properly applies only to a peripheral to central chaining theory and not one in which associations involve only central representations.

here of the wide range of skills, species, and methods over which movement persists following feedback removal.

Wilson (1961) in a now classic study severed the nerves that return feedback from wingbeats in the locust. Although the rate of beating slowed, the beat pattern was largely maintained, suggesting central rather than peripheral control. The vocal system of birds is innervated bilaterally by the hypoglossal nerve. When one side of the nerve or the other is severed, paralyzing the muscles on the denervated side, portions of the bird's song drop out (Nottebohm, 1970). The remaining elements of the song occur in the proper time slots, however, demon-strating that neither the missing kinesthetic feedback nor the missing auditory feedback from the eliminated segments is needed for triggering the remaining segments. Again S-R chaining theory appears ruled out, since the proper se-quence of movements is maintained in the absence of some portions of the feedback. Related phenomena have been demonstrated in mammals as well. During grooming a normal mouse brings its forepaws in front of its face, and as the paws move toward the mouth, the tongue licks out and makes contact with the paws. In another sequence one forelimb crosses over the eye, and the eye closes just before contact. Fentress (1973a) amputated the forelimbs of mice at 1 day of age. Grooming behaviors were observed up to 30 days of age even though they no longer could serve a grooming function. The remaining portions of the limbs in the amputated mice went through the same grooming motions shown by normal mice and the tongue licked or the eye closed at the appro-priate time even though no forepaw contact with the face was possible and all sources of feedback from that missing segment was lost. Apparently the move-ment sequence is inborn, since amputation occurred at one day, and its proper execution does not depend on the tactual, kinesthetic, or other feedback from the missing limb.

The control of movement by locusts, birds and mice may be far different from the skills of humans, however. For that reason, the experiments with perhaps the greatest impact on our thinking about human skills involved rhesus monkeys. Taub and Berman (1968) repeated a historic experiment by Mott and Sherring-ton (1895). Kinesthetic feedback was surgically eliminated from one of the monkey's front legs by severing the dorsal roots of the nerve bundles entering the spinal cord, eliminating the afferent feedback but not influencing the efferent input to the muscles.

As observed by Mott and Sherrington, monkeys avoided using the single deafferented limb. Historically, observations of this sort led to S-R chaining theory. Taub and Berman further observed, however, that restraining the normal forelimb encouraged the animal to use the deafferented one. Moreover, when both forelimbs were deafferented, ". . . the animals were able to use the limbs rhythmically and in excellent coordination with the hind limbs during slow and even moderately fast ambulation [p. 177] ." The monkeys could also climb wire cages, and walking and climbing persisted with blindfolding in addition to deafferentation. More recently, Taub et al. (1973) demonstrated that infant monkeys both deafferented and visually blocked shortly after birth learn to walk, suggesting that the sequence of movements underlying walking does not depend on normal, detailed feedback for the development of the skill.

Criticisms of the Taub and Berman study have been raised on at least three points. The first two suggest that some kinesthetic feedback may have remained. One argument is that all afferents in the dorsal roots may not have been severed during the surgical procedure. As one guard against this possibility, Taub and Berman stimulated the nerve ends in the deafferented limb and observed no evoked cortical responses. Evoked potentials might be expected if some kinesthetic sense remained. Bossom and Ommaya (1968) also confirmed that monkeys could both walk and grasp objects when deafferentation was done with more precise microscopic surgery, making it more likely that all the desired dorsal afferents were cut. Second, a small proportion of the kinesthetic afferents may enter the spinal cord through the ventral roots rather than the severed dorsal roots (Bossom, 1974). The fact that Taub and Berman did not observe cortical evoked potentials to nerve stimulation and that Bossom and Ommaya found no reflex responses to pin pricks or pinching is some evidence, though not conclusive, that no functional kinesthetic sense remains after dorsal root deafferentation. Nevertheless, some reservation must be maintained about the Taub and Berman study if some afferents do enter the ventral roots. At the same time, however, the procedures of the Nottebohm and Fentress studies are not susceptible to the same criticisms, since some segments of the movement series were eliminated entirely. Although those studies do deal with lower animals, they lead to the same conclusion.

A third, more serious issue has been raised by Bossom (1974). Whereas Taub and Berman emphasize the high degree of coordination in walking that monkeys retain following deafferentation, Bossom emphasizes the loss of elegance of movement control. Much recovery occurs following extensive postsurgical practice. The monkeys can, for example, extend their arms, bend their wrists, and curl their fingers around a food object, even when the arm is hidden from view. Apparently, however, the thumb is not used in such movements, and movements generally appear clumsy. It is possible that the more gross rhythmic movements involved in skills like walking can be sequenced without feedback, but that finer manipulative skills or more distal skills are dependent on feedback. If such is the case, it does not necessarily mean that feedback is a required stimulus for succeeding movements as in S-R chaining theory. Instead, the feedback may be necessary for either finer or more frequent corrections in the skill the finer the task required. Alternatively, the skills for which the motor program concept best apply may have a strong innate component. Manipualtive skills may be primarily learned, and the mode of representation may be different.

As a whole these studies suggest that the sequence of movements in at least some skills is centrally represented as a motor program An appropriate sequence of neural commands can be sent to the muscles, resulting in the desired movement, even though no feedback unique to individual movements returns from the periphery to stimulate successive movements. The motor program concept does not imply that feedback is not an extremely important element of skilled performance. It is. Furthermore, the existence of motor programs does not imply that S-R chaining is not also possible. Both mechanisms may coexist or apply to different skills. As mentioned, the skills on which the motor program concept are based have a strong innate component. Many human skills, on the other hand, are learned skills, and for that type of skill virtually no evidence exists on the form of representation. S-R chaining theory essentially is a learning theory, not a theory of innate representation, and it may therefore fare better for learned skills.

Evidence for motor programs in humans is less adequate than for animals because of the difficulty of manipulating kinesthetic sensations without permanent neural damage. One promising technique, explored by Lazlo (1966, 1967), uses a pressure cuff on the upper arm to block blood flow to the lower arm. Lazlo claimed that following cuff application, people lost their kinesthetic sensation prior to deficits in motor functions. Despite kinesthetic loss, people were able to tap their fingers, though at a reduced rate, even with blindfolds and auditory masking noise. Although some studies found greater deficits on more complex skills (for a review, see Glencross, 1975), Docherty (1973) demonstrated that a finger sequencing task could be performed fairly well under kinesthetic block.

Unfortunately, conclusions from studies using pressure blocks face severe interpretive problems. Glencross (1975) reported that people are able to perceive elbow and wrist movement when finger sensation is lost. Remaining sensory information perhaps could be used for performing the sequential task, especially since many of the muscles that operate the fingers are in the forearm where sensory cutoff appears less complete. On the other hand, Kelso et al. (1974) applied supramaximal electric shocks to the skin overlaying the median and ulnar nerves and above the point of application of the pressure cuff. Since the stimulation is supramaximal, any changes in evoked muscle responses cannot be ascribed to inadequate stimulation. Both the latency and amplitude of evoked muscle responses below the cuff exhibited considerable decrement before sensory perception disappeared completely. Thus, when decrements occur on tasks following cuff application, it may reflect motor impairment, not sensory loss. At this point, therefore, the kinesthetic block technique appears unanalytic.

Another approach for studying kinesthetic loss in humans is to observe people who have had dorsal roots cut to control pain or relieve spasticity. Although the operation has been done many times, there appear to be few studies of the motor consequences. Foerster (reported in Phillips, 1969) in the early 1900s found that patients with deafferentation of arms and hands could move them as directed, even without vision. As with monkeys, however, much fine control of the fingers was lost, and patients had difficulty moving individual fingers without moving others at the same time. Perhaps motor programs are involved to a greater extent in gross limb movements than in fine movements or finger movements or in sequential skills instead of isolated finger movements, but critical tests have not been conducted. One might ask, for example, whether highly practiced sequential skills such as typing can be executed with the fingers following deafferentation. Tasks involving isolated movements such as an animal plucking an object between thumb and forefinger or a person moving a particular finger may be difficult following deafferentation because such tasks do not involve highly predictable and sequential skills. By their nature they may be dependent on feedback, but other sequential finger skills might be more free.

In general, therefore, observations following deafferentation in humans are consistent with those of animals but not as conclusive. At least some simple movements appear to be made without kinesthetic feedback, ruling out S-R chaining theory as a necessary component. Again, however, evidence is lacking on the form of representation for more complex learned skills. The relative lack of evidence of the form of representation for learned skills requires caution. Nevertheless, it is useful to pursue the possible implications that motor program theory has for human learning, and this will be done later.

A. Follow-Up Servo Theory and Alpha-Gamma Coactivation Theories

Two predominant theories have been proposed regarding how a central representation is translated into the appropriate muscular movement. Both theories involve the gamma-efferent kinesthetic system.[2] Follow-up servo theory, discussed by Matthews (1964) and Phillips (1969), imparts a critical role to the gamma system in actually causing muscular movement. Alpha-gamma coactivation theory postulates parallel programming of both the gamma efferents and the main muscle system; the gamma system senses errors but is not critical in actually implementing movement.

The gamma system, often called the fusimotor system, has a unique property of adjustable sensitivity. Embedded within the main muscles are stretch receptors called muscle spindle receptors. If a main muscle is passively stretched, a spindle receptor embedded in the muscle is likewise stretched and the neural output from that receptor increases. The spindle receptor is also connected to its

---

[2] A more detailed description of the gamma system and other kinesthetic senses is given in many sources on neurophysiology. Two good sources are Howard and Templeton (1966) and Matthews (1964). In the present context only very general features of the gamma efferent system are described.

own unique muscle fiber, called an intrafusal fiber, and that fiber can be programmed independently of the main muscle by the gamma efferents. Alpha efferents innervate the extrafusal fibers of the main muscles. The intrafusal fibers, when activated by gamma efferents, are unable to move limbs, but they do control the degree of stretch in the spindle independently of the passive stretch caused by coupling to the main muscle. Furthermore, some of the afferent neurons that return feedback from the stretch receptor also make synaptic connections in the spinal cord with the alpha motoneurons that activate the main muscles. The fusimotor system, therefore, is one that can be directly programmed itself, but it is also passively influenced by the muscles to which it is coupled.

In follow-up servo theory, the central nervous system programs the gamma neurons rather than the alpha motoneurons. Activation of gamma neurons contracts the spindles. Spindle receptors are therefore stretched, resulting in increased neural discharge, and that discharge feeds back on the alpha motoneurons. The alpha motoneurons in turn activate the main muscle, and the limb moves. As the main muscle contracts, stretch on the muscle spindle declines until the receptor output returns to baseline. At that point the output from the muscle spindle no longer facilitates the alpha neurons, so the main muscle stops contracting. Thus, the spindle system is programmed by the gamma efferents, and the main muscle reflexively follows until it nulls out the programmed stretch of the muscle spindles.

The follow-up servo notion appears at first unduly complicated, since the central nervous system presumably could directly program the alpha motoneurons going to the main muscles and hence eliminate the servo loop, but some reflection reveals attractive features of a follow-up servo. One perplexing observation about motor skills is that the same task is seldom if ever performed twice in exactly the same way. How can motor program theory explain such a result? If the system programs spindle settings, then the main muscles would be driven by the reflex loop to the desired position in space even though the starting position varies from trial to trial. Furthermore, spindle settings often may be changed before the servo loop has completed its operation. Thus, at the level of programming there could be a great deal of stereotypy in the sense of spindle settings, but the actual movement could exhibit much variability on different occasions.

A very similar point has been made by MacNeilage (1970) and Sussman (1972) regarding speech production. The same phoneme is acoustically different in the context of different surrounding phonemes. Moreover, the required movement for the tongue to reach a position desired for the production of a particular phoneme depends on the tongue's preceding position, which is, of course, different for different preceding phonemes. Must the brain store a motor program for every combination of phonemes? MacNeilage and Sussman propose instead that muscle spindles, not movements, are programmed and the movement is reflexively driven by the spindle system. Thus, the programming is context free even though the output varies with context. A servo system would, therefore, offer some economy in the flexibility of programming.

At this point the question may be raised whether follow-up servo theory is not the same as S-R chaining theory and whether it has not already been discounted by deafferentation studies. The two theories are, in fact, quite different. In S-R chaining theory, one movement is stimulated by the feedback from a preceding movement. If feedback from the preceding movement is eliminated or the preceding movement is eliminated altogether, the chain is broken. The studies of Fentress on mouse grooming and Nottebohm on birdsong discount S-R chaining theory because the remainder of a sequence is not broken when parts of a sequence are lost. With follow-up servo theory, however, the movement is centrally programmed and does not require feedback from a prior movement; it only requires feedback from the muscle spindles associated with the current movement.

The deafferentation studies of Taub and Berman and of Foerster pose greater problems for follow-up servo theory. If there are no spindle connections from an intact limb into the spinal cord and onto the alpha motoneurons (i.e., if the dorsal roots are cut), then no coordinated movement should occur. Coordinated movement does occur, however, seemingly rejecting servo theory. It is worthwhile to recall, though, that deafferentation has more serious consequences for fine movements than gross ones. Perhaps servo mechanisms are more important the finer the degree of movement control such as by hand or tongue. This issue will be returned to shortly.

Alpha-gamma coactivation theory bears some similarity to follow-up servo theory, but in principle it accomodates movement following deafferentation. In this theory, the two efferent systems are programmed in parallel. The motor program sends commands via the alpha route to activate the main muscles in the desired sequence and via the gamma system to activate the muscle spindles. Matthews (1964) and Phillips (1969) propose that this parallel system allows rapid error corrections but at the same time avoids extra starting time for movements entailed by follow-up servo theories.

Suppose, to simplify the argument, the motor program stimulates the muscle spindle via the gamma system to exactly compensate for movement of the main muscle. As the extrafusal fibers of the main muscle contract and shorten, they tend to release tension on the stretch receptor, but simultaneously the gamma system activates the intrafusal fiber counteracting the influence of the main muscle. When the two systems exactly counterbalance, no change will occur in receptor stretch and consequently the receptor discharge will remain constant. If, however, the moving limb encounters an unexpected force, the extrafusal fiber will not contract as much as it should, because extrafusal fibers are connected to the bones and if the bones are prevented from moving, the extrafusal fibers are prevented from contracting. The intrafusal fiber, not being connected to the impeded bone structure, will continue contracting as programmed. The balance of forces on the stretch receptor will be lost and it will stretch, increasing in discharge and signaling that an unexpected impediment occurred. Because feedback returns to the alpha system it can act reflexively at either the spinal level or higher brain levels to boost input to the alpha motoneurons and overcome the unexpected impediment. Marsden *et al.* (1972) found corrective responses, presumably dependent on stretch receptors, to occur in human thumb movement about 50 msec following an unexpected force. At the same time Evarts and Tanji (1974) have shown that the reflex is capable of presetting so that an unexpected force can be countered with either a push or a pull, depending on prior instruction. This suggests that corrective action occurs at brain levels or brain functions can preset spinal reflexes by descending control.

Thus, alpha-gamma coactivation preserves some of the advantage of follow-up servo theory. It has a mechanism for fast compensation to unexpected forces, driving the limb by a servo mechanism to the desired position. But because alpha motoneurons are independently programmed, sequencing of movements can still occur following deafferentation, though the error correction capability would be lost.

B. Evidence Discriminating between the Two Theories

Both follow-up servo theory and alpha-gamma coactivation theory posit active programming of the spindle system predicting that spindle output should either increase or at least remain constant during active movement. If, on the other hand, the spindle receptor only responds passively to stretch of the main muscles, and is not itself programmed, the spindle output should decrease as the main muscles contract and reduce the stretch. One suitable preparation for studying whether spindle output increases, stays constant, or decreases during active movement is the intercostal muscles involved in breathing. The intercostal muscles are useful because a regular movement pattern is maintained even when the animal is anesthetized and immobilized. Von Euler (1965) found in cats that as the intercostal muscles contract, forcing air out of the lungs, firing rate from the muscle spindles increases, as predicted by active programming of the muscle spindles. Moreover, if during the course of breathing an unexpected load is placed on the intercostal muscles by temporarily occluding the windpipe and creating a partial vacuum to retard further muscle contraction, the spindle output is increased even further. This increased output to unexpected loads is exactly the sort of error correction expected by either theory.

A very similar phenomenon was observed by Taylor and Cody (1974) for movements of the jaw in licking and eating by cats. Whereas spindle output varied as a function of main muscle stretch during passive jaw movements, spindle output remained practically constant during self-generated licking, indicating active programming of the muscle spindle. The fact that output remained constant supports alpha-gamma coactivation.

A necessary implication of follow-up servo theory is that the gamma system must become active before the alpha system and the main muscles, since the alpha system is activated by the feedback from the gamma loop. Historically, studies indicated that the gamma system leads the alpha system but those studies involved animals under deep anesthesia. Apparently anesthesia can alter the time relationships of alpha and gamma. Phillips (1969) with his colleagues Koeze and Sheridan studied muscle responses from the hand of the baboon under light anesthesia that more closely approximates the normal state. They elicited the muscle responses by electrical pulses to the cortex and observed the onset times of the electromyographic response from the muscle and the discharge from muscle spindles recorded at the dorsal roots. Under some conditions they found spindle discharge to increase during muscle contraction. As with Euler's study of breathing movements and Taylor and Cody's study of jaw movements, this finding indicates active programming of the muscle spindles, since muscle contraction by itself would lead to a decrease in spindle output. In addition, the spindle discharge in some circumstances occurred at the same time as or followed the muscle response, indicating that the gamma system is not activated early enough for its discharge to feedback on and start the main muscles. This study therefore rules out follow-up servo theory and supports the theory of alpha-gamma coactivation.

Even more convincing evidence comes from a study by Vallbo (1971) of voluntary muscle contractions by people. He inserted an electrode into the median nerve of the arm and located responses from a single afferent fiber from a muscle spindle. Subjects in the experiment were then asked either to flex a finger for 2 or more seconds or twitch the finger. In either case a large proportion of spindle responses followed, rather than preceded, activation of the muscle underlying finger movement. Again this supports alpha-gamma coactivation theory.

The studies of the activation and timing of the spindle system are, therefore, consistent with deafferentation studies. Some movements are programmable directly through the alpha system to the main muscles without feedback from the spindle system. Some cautions are worth holding in mind, however. Neither Phillips' study of the baboon hand nor Vallbo's study of finger movement, the two studies most critical for differentiating the two theories, involved sequential movement skills. All they demonstrated is that movements can start without a follow-up servo mechanism, but they have little to say about whether terminal movement points are also programmed through the alpha system. There is some provocative evidence that the gamma system or other feedback sources are more directly involved in finely controlled movements after they have started.

Smith *et al.* (1972) attempted to selectively anesthetize gamma fibers by injecting Xylocaine in the radial nerve. The gamma fibers are small in diameter compared to alpha fibers. Under the right dosage, the small fibers appear blocked, since hot and cold stimulation which also involves small fibers is not perceived. At the same time, strength and tactile sensations subserved by large fibers are normal. This suggests that alpha fibers are also intact. In one task following selective blocking of small fibers, subjects were asked to rapidly touch their noses. Normally one observes a slight pause just before touching the nose, but people with gamma blocking failed to stop their fingers on the first couple of tries and instead forcefully hit their cheeks or mouths, as though the feedback was needed for stopping the movement. Although they were soon able to overcome this failure to stop, the results raise the possibility that the gamma system is normally involved in terminating movements. Other interpretations, such as some motor impairment, are possible, however.

Evidence of a similar sort comes from Bizzi's studies (1974) of eye and head movements in monkeys. Normally when a spot of light comes on in the periphery of the visual field, the eyes make a saccadic jump to fixate on the spot. Very soon after the eyes begin moving, the head also begins to turn toward the source; as the head rotates, the eyes make a compensatory back turn in the sockets. Eventually the head is pointing at the spot, and the eyes are again pointing straight ahead in their sockets. When vestibular feedback was surgically interrupted, eye and head movements were both initiated but compensatory eye movement failed to occur; apparently that final phase of compensatory movement was reflex controlled. With several weeks of training, compensatory movement did recover, perhaps then under complete central control. Like Smith *et al.*, Bizzi appears to have uncovered a movement sequence that is initiated by program, but the termination normally is partly under feedback control, in this case vestibular feedback.

A final behavioral study is of interest in this context. Stelmach *et al.* (1975) required people to rapidly move a slider to a position along a track, remove their arm momentarily, and then recall the same ending location by moving from a different starting position. In one condition the first movement of the pair was determined by the subject himself. Since the movement was rapid, the subject presumably selected the stopping location prior to beginning the movement. In two other conditions, the subject's hand was either passively moved to a location matched to positions in the preselection case or the subject actively moved until hitting a stop at the location. In neither of the latter cases did the subject know in advance where he would stop. At the final stopping position, subjects in all conditions held position for 2 sec. Despite this end pause, preselection subjects were more accurate in reproducing the location. Why?

There are perhaps several possibilities, but an intriguing one is that only the preselection condition allows advance programming of the movement. But programming of movement distance is not possible in this situation since the subjects reproduce location. Perhaps it is the muscle spindles that are set for a final location and are remembered during reproduction. If so, then the finding would constitute evidence that spindles are intimately involved in precise movement termination.

Although the bulk of evidence supports a motor programming theory involving alpha-gamma coactivation, these latter studies, while far from conclusive, raise the possibility that a hybrid between the coactivation and follow-up servo mechanisms might be involved. Perhaps the alpha system conveys programs for the initiation of movements and even their rough termination. Parallel with the initiation of movements through the alpha route, spindles may be coactivated. While they may not be necessary for starting the movement, they may come into play, as supposed by follow-up servo theory, in finely graded movement termination. Again, the fusimotor system may not be absolutely necessary for ending movements, but it may aid such termination and make it more precise. Coactivation theory, in contrast, gives the gamma system a role only in correcting errors and not in the normal stopping of movement. Such a hybrid system would include all the advantages of the follow-up servo theory, including partial explanation of context dependent variations in movement, but also would be consistent with rapid starting of movements, the persistence of movements following deafferentation, and coactivation of alpha and gamma. Such a hybrid model is similar to a servo-assisted model proposed by Merton (1972) but is only speculative at this time as evidence is suggestive but definitely not conclusive.

The main conclusion to draw at this point is that at least some skills appear under motor program control. Some skills are directly programmed through the alpha route, but subsidiary programming may also occur through the gamma route resulting in more precise movement termination. Yet other skills may not be under program control. Thus, we do not know whether finer skills or skills performed by distal elements such as the fingers are programmed, since they are disrupted more by loss of feedback; they could be programmed, but feedback is needed for more frequent correction, or feedback may actually be needed for initiating movements as supposed by S-R chaining or closed-loop conceptions of skill.

C. General Functions of Feedback

At this point it is useful to broaden the discussion to other feedback sources to gain a fuller perspective on the interaction between program and feedback in skill development and maintenance. A very instructive skill for this perspective is birdsong. Bird species that have been most useful in studying skill development are ones exhibiting some flexibility in song development such as the Oregon Junco, White-crowned Sparrow, and European Chaffinch. In normal development young birds are exposed to adult singing in about the first 4 months of life and begin to sing themselves at about 10 months of age. Nottebohm (1970) and others report that the young nestling can be exposed to adult song either in nature or in the laboratory in those first 4 months, and even when isolated for the remaining months, it will learn the proper dialect. In contrast, birds that are not exposed at all to the adult song learn only a rudimentary version. The young birds must, therefore, store in memory a template of the auditory sound pattern in order to subsequently learn the song.

Building on preliminary observations of this type, Konishi (1965) exposed young birds to adult song so that a template was stored. Some birds were then deafened prior to learning to sing themselves. Their subsequent song development was even more impaired than for birds never exposed to an adult song, but at least able to hear themselves. On the other hand, if deafening was delayed until the song was firmly established, the song remained remarkably stable. Konishi found the song of one White-crowned Sparrow to persist very well for at least 18 months after deafening.

The model of skill learning and maintenance that emerges both from the studies of birdsong and the numerous studies underlying the motor program concept is illustrated in Figure 2. One component of the skill is a template or

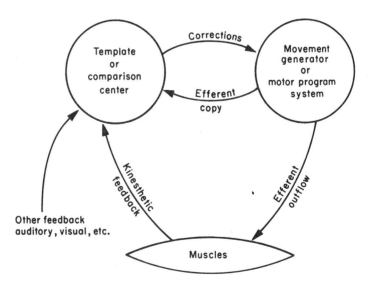

Figure 2 A model of skill learning and a mechanism for the detection and correction of errors.

model of how the feedback should appear if the skill is properly performed. In birdsong an auditory template is emphasized, but conceptually in other cases a template could as well include visual and kinesthetic components.[3] A motor program center generates a series of movements via efferent outflow to the muscles. The movements generate kinesthetic feedback from the limbs and the movements have a variety of other sensory consequences—auditory, visual, and vestibular—depending on the skill. The feedback is then matched to the template, and any resultant error leads to correction of the motor program. Eventually the program will emit an appropriate series of movements, and the program with further practice becomes stabilized.

This model of skill learning is similar in many respects to a theory of Adams (1971). In Adams' theory, feedback is also compared to a template of ideal feedback established during training, and deviations of current feedback from the template are the basis for corrections.

If the environment in which a skill is performed is very stable or predictable, the feedback loop can be cut and the skill can be maintained by the program. With birds, once the song is well learned the auditory feedback can be eliminated (Konishi, 1965) and at least parts of the kinesthetic feedback can be eliminated (Nottebohm, 1970) with little or no song impairment. If the skill is robust it may still be fairly well maintained with greatly impoverished feedback even in a varying environment. Monkeys, for example, walk on four legs, a relatively stable stance, so that the skill persists rather well following deafferentation and blindfolding.

For many human skills, however, the environment is less than perfectly predictable and the skill itself may be imperfectly executed so that error constantly arises. Feedback cannot then be eliminated; it is continually needed for monitoring the movement to ensure that performance is progressing as planned and for updating or changing programs as needed (Pew, 1974). But in the absence of a need for correction, the feedback does not stimulate the succeeding movement as posited by S-R chaining theory. The model in Figure 2 thus presents a combination of closed-loop and open-loop capability.

Many people have noted a tremendous difference between the highly stereotyped skills of birdsong and walking by monkeys and the great degree of flexibility of human skill. Human skills seldom are executed in exactly the same way twice. The movement can be large or small—one's handwriting on the blackboard is similar to handwriting with paper and pencil despite enormous differences in the muscles involved—there are differences in speed, exact sequencing, orientation, and so on. Although these observations pose as yet unsolved

---

[3] There may be important properties of an auditory template, however, and that is an idea well worth exploring in skill learning. Auditory patterns coupled with movement patterns permits real time feedback, and audition may be better than vision for displaying temporal patterns.

problems for understanding skills, they are not necessarily inconsistent with motor program theory; the theory as specified just does not go far enough for a complete understanding of these problem. The problems posed for S-R chaining are more serious. When the actual muscles involved dramatically change from one performance of a skill to another, the feedback is also changed. Previously unexperienced feedback patterns should result in skill breakdown, since that feedback would not be conditioned to the next response. Motor program theory stripped to its essentials, in contrast, merely proposes that the sequencing of movements is centrally generated and does not directly depend on prior feedback for its execution. Exactly how the sequencing is determined is unspecified.

Some conceptual advances in understanding the knotty problem of skill variation have been made by Pew (1974) and Schmidt (1975). Both have suggested that motor programs do not directly specify either a series of specific muscle movements or expectations for particular feedback. Rather they are best viewed as a schema of possible movements and expected feedback. In the context of a particular situation, parameters such as speed, size, orientation, and so on are applied to the schema to generate a particular sequence of movement. At the same time the schema generates a set of expected feedback consequences (the template) that should arise if the skill is performed as specified. Schmidt (1975) has fleshed out many details of a schema conception of motor programs. For the present chapter, however, it is sufficient to view a motor program as a central representation of a motor sequence that can in the absence of error be initiated and carried out without subsequent stimulation from kinesthetic feedback. At this simplistic level, the model portrayed in Figure 2 has implications for skill learning, and it raises various psychological issues regarding the nature of representation.

D. Implications for Skill Learning

Loop films and video feedback have both been heavily investigated as aids to skill learning. With loop films, the technique of a highly skilled performer is shown many times to a learner. The learner then tries to copy the performance of the model. Video feedback involves the use of movies or video tape recordings to play back the learner's own performance so that he can observe the errors he has made and presumably correct them. It appears fair to say that neither technique has proved highly useful in skill training. Brumbach (1969) reviewed 31 studies that used one or the other technique as a teaching aid. Of those only 10 indicated that films were helpful, but as Brumbach pointed out, 5 of those 10 studies had serious problems such as no data shown, no statistical tests, etc. Three of the remaining five had mixed results favoring the use of films.

One possible reason for such a dismal failure is that most studies used only loop films and a few used only video feedback. Only 4 of the 31 studies used both techniques together and 3 of those 4 were among the studies showing an advantage of film techniques over control training procedures. The model of skill learning shown in Figure 2 indicates two general components involved in skill learning. One is the template, i.e., memory for what the feedback should be like when the skill is properly performed. The other component is the actual feedback generated from execution of the motor program. Learning with a loop film provides a template but inadequate feedback to complete the learning loop. Since people have a difficult time visualizing the movements of their body, the situation is not unlike a bird with an auditory template but deaf so that it is unable to compare its own performance to the template. Learning with only video feedback presents the opposite problem; there is an inadequate model for comparison with the feedback. Figure 2 suggests that the most effective skill learning requires a careful match of the feedback provided to the template stored. Usually no emphasis is given to the quality of the match between two sources of information, and this principle might be useful in investigating training procedures.

Although feedback is an essential component of skill learning, sometimes portions of the feedback can be dropped once they have served the role of establishing the proper movement sequence. In birdsong auditory feedback is critical during learning but not essential once the movement pattern is well established. This implication is quite different than would be expected from strictly closed-loop theories of skill such as S-R chaining.

In cases where natural sources of feedback are impoverished, therefore, it may prove useful to temporarily provide artificial feedback merely for purposes of learning. For example, movements in some skills could be coupled to sound transducers to provide an auditory sound pattern that varies with the movement and that can be compared with sound patterns produced by experts. Once the skill is learned, the auditory feedback can be dropped. A possible advantage of this technique is that auditory feedback can be provided in real time whereas video feedback often can be provided only after the skill is performed. The auditory feedback may also provide the learner with a greater appreciation of the temporal aspects of the skill.

Two research programs on speech production attempted to exploit the possible benefit of feedback substitution in cases where natural feedback is inadequate. One involved learning a foreign language and the other, still in progress, involves speech training in the deaf.

A prevalent problem in learning a second language is that some important sound distinctions in the new language are difficult to perceive, and this handicap impairs pronunciation learning. To help overcome the problem, Kalikow and Rollins (1973) and Kalikow (1974) extracted various acoustic features and throat vibrations from spoken words and visually displayed transformations of them on an oscilloscope screen. In Mandarin Chinese, the tone quality arising from variations in the fundamental voice frequency is a determinant of meaning. Contours of the fundamental frequency as it changes within a syllabic or multisyllabic utterance can be displayed on the scope. By presenting transformations of a teacher's utterance and a student's utterance next to each other, the student receives cues on how to improve pronunciation. Kalikow found in comparison to control groups without the aids that the visual system modestly improved pronunciation of both Mandarin Chinese by native English speakers and English by Spanish speakers. Unfortunately, with the current development of the system it is not yet clear that the modest improvement is worthwhile from either economic or student-time viewpoints.

Nearly the same system is being explored by Nickerson and Stevens (1973) to train the deaf to speak. Again, visual displays present transformations of the learner's speech to be compared with a model. As yet, results from this project are not available. Nonetheless, in view of the modest success with second language learning, better achievement might be expected with the deaf, since their natural feedback from speaking is even more imporverished.

An implication of S-R theory is that the skill must be executed for learning to occur, for only in that way will kinesthetic feedback be available for conditioning to succeeding movements. Figure 2 suggests instead that important components of the skill may be learned without actual movement production. One component is an accurate template of desired feedback. As with birdsong, sometimes the template may be established prior to learning movements. This may be the procedure underlying the outstanding success of the Suzuki method of violin teaching (Pronko, 1969). In the Suzuki method very young children are exposed to selected pieces of music, sometimes for months or years, prior to actually handling an instrument. Perhaps the detailed music templates that the children store in memory allow them to subsequently recognize errors in their own sound production and later the sequencing of movements that lead to the sound.

Besides storing a template without actual movement, it also may be possible to store part of the motor program itself. Mental practice is known to improve performance on many skills (e.g., Lawther, 1968). What is the explanation? A central element of motor program theory, is that it represents sequences of successive movements. Any skill in which sequencing is a major component might be helped by mentally rehearsing the sequence of environmental events or required movements until the sequence is firmly stored in the memory system. Summers (1973) tested this idea in a study consisting primarily of responding as rapidly as possible to events that tend to occur in sequential order. Rehearsal of the event order was effective even when movements were not used until later in the task.

Motor program theory suggests several ways, therefore, in which skill training might be improved. It suggests that the quality of the match between feedback and model is critical. It suggests that temporary provision of artificial feedback may be useful, particularly when it can be matched with a comparable model. In some instances the establishment of feedback templates prior to actual movement practice may be beneficial. In other circumstances, mental rehearsal of the sequence of events may be useful.

III. Memory Structures of Motor Programs

Granted that movement sequences in skills often are centrally represented, how do we conceptualize the memory structure? Is the program a chain of associations between central representations of the movements or are successive movements associated not one with the other but with positions in a more abstract structure? For movement sequences exhibiting a high order of regularity, are the movements stored in the form of generative rules? We would also like to know how the timing of motor skills is meshed with the sequence representation. These are the issues addressed in this final section.

A. Simple Movement Structures

One approach to the problem of representation was investigated by Keele (1975). To capture in abstract form the sequential property of many skills, a task was developed in which sequencing was the primary component. There were eight lights in a horizontal line and beneath the lights was a row of response keys, one key for each light. When a light appeared, the subject pressed the corresponding key, extinguishing the light. Another light requiring a response then came on, and so on. During the initial training the lights appeared in a recurring order. If the lights are designated 1 through 8 from left to right, the order of occurrence for all subjects was 18347562 after which it cycled back to 1 with no break. This task is much like playing a piano or typing with the exceptions that it is simpler, very easy to learn, and cycles repetitively through the sequence much as does walking. Within a half-hour subjects can execute the series at rapid speeds.

Once the skill is well imprinted in memory, how is it represented? Two possibilities were compared by examining response times when the proper order of events was momentarily disrupted and then restarted. One possible representation, event-to-event associations, posits that successive movements are associated with each other. The other hypothesis, event-to-position associations, posits that movements are not associated one with the other but with positions in the sequence.

To obtain a better idea what these hypotheses mean, consider the experimental situation. Suppose a subject is presented sequentially with lights 3475,

```
1 8 3 4 7 5 6 2 . . .        Normal sequence

1 8 3 4 7 5 8 . . .          The last event 8 is out of order

1 8 3 4 7 5 8 3 . . .        Event association (3 normally follows 8)

1 8 3 4 7 5 8 2 . . .        Position association (2 is in its normal
                                                       position)
```

Figure 3 Examples of restarting a sequence of events following an out-of-order event for subjects assigned to the Event Association group and for subjects assigned to the Position Association group.

which are in correct order, and the next light is out of order and is light 8 (recall that the complete correct sequence is 18347562; see Figure 3). Because light 8 is unexpected, people are slow in responding to it. Now there are at least two interesting ways for the sequence to restart following an unexpected event. In the one case the very next light is 3, the one that normally follows light 8. The hypothetical sequence then is 3475834 . . . and so on till the next out of order event. In the second case, light 2 follows 8, so the hypothetical sequence would be 3475821 . . . until the next light out of order. The unexpected event 8 replaces the expected event 6 but subsequent events occur in their proper positions. Light 2 is normally the second light after 5 regardless of which light intervened. In the first case, therefore, an event is predictable by the preceding event, even though the preceding event itself may be out of order. In the second case, an event is predictable by the position in sequence regardless of what the preceding event was.

The issue, of course, is how well people can respond to the first event back in sequence. If the return to sequence is predicted by events, then people should respond rapidly to the first event back in sequence only if the memory structure consists of event-to-event associations. On the other hand, if the return is predicted by position, people should do well only if the memory structure consists of event-to-position associations.

People in the experiment received training on the cyclical sequence until they could respond rapidly and the skill presumably was well set in memory. On the next day the task remained about the same, but people were told that 20% of the lights would be out of the expected order, and following such an intrusion the sequence would restart. For half the people the event succeeding an out of order one was predicted by the identity of the out of order event. For the other half, the event succeeding the out of order one was predicted by the position in the sequence. An additional variable was the interval between one response and the next light. With a relatively long interval (1500 msec RSI), allowing ample time for anticipation of the following light, it was expected that people could effectively use either type of sequence return. But at short response-stimulus intervals (50 msec RSI) people might experience difficulty in using one type or the other of sequence return.

Reaction times are shown in Figure 4 for unexpected lights, designated the 0 position in the sequence, and for the first, second, third, and fourth lights back in sequence. Although people in the position condition respond slightly faster on the average when a long RSI allows ample time for preparation, they are slower than event condition subjects at the short RSI. In other words, when the subjects are pressed for time, they are unable to effectively use position information, but use of event information suffers little. The improvement in reaction time from the unexpected event to the first back in sequence is a measure of preparation for the succeeding event. At the long RSI both conditions show an improvement on the order of 160 msec. However, at the short RSI, when spare time is not available, people in the event condition again show a large improvement but people in the position condition show very little improvement. The modest improvement that does occur in the latter case is probably in part an artifact: If two successive unexpected events occur, the second one is usually responded to faster than the first as though the unexpected is no longer surprising. When time is short, an event predictable by position is little or no better, therefore, than another unpredictable event.

Our results suggest that in some skills a sequence of events and their corresponding movements are stored in a chain of event-to-event associations. This conclusion is very much in line with the theoretical position of Wickelgren (1969), though he was primarily concerned with the phonetic representation of words. A classic paper by Lashley (1951) suggested in contrast that the memory structure of serial order is independent of the actual events that fit into the

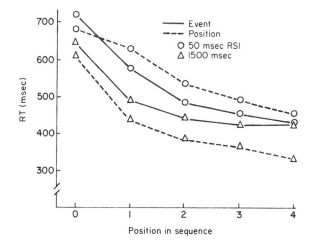

Figure 4 Mean reaction time to correct responses for out-of-sequence events (○) and the first, second, third, and fourth events back in sequence. The interval between a response and the next stimulus is short (50 msec) or long (1000 msec).

structure. A position structure of the sort investigated in this study would be an example of a structure other than event associations but by no means the only possible one. According to the position conception, the skill is represented as a number of slots, one for each movement. As the skill progresses, one slot after the other is examined for content, and the event or movement contained in the slot is prepared for. Preparation for a movement depends not on the preceding event but only on the current position. A position stepping structure is not supported by this experiment, but in other skills with structural regularities, a representation that is neither event associations or purely position associations may be indicated. This point will be returned to later.

The preceding experiment does not support the position hypothesis as out-lined, but with other assumptions the position theory might be accommodated to the data. For example, when an unexpected event occurs, a position marker might skip forward in the sequence until the position of the unexpected event is found. According to this view a position hypothesis would make the same prediction as the event association hypothesis for the preceding data. The next experiment dealing with repeated elements was therefore designed as a further test between the two theories.

A conceptual problem faced by the event-to-event hypothesis concerns re-peated elements. If the identical movement occurs at more than one place in a movement sequence, and each time it is followed by a different movement, then how are simple one-to-one assocations able to determine what movement should follow the repeated one? In typing, if the letter H follows the letter T in one position and E follows T in another position, how does the typist know whether to type H or E following a T if only event associations are used. Associational hypotheses might be elaborated in several ways to handle this problem. Wickel-gren (1969), for example, proposed that seemingly identical elements in differ-ent portions of a sequence in fact are not identical and differ slightly depending on their surrounding movements.[4] Nevertheless, repeated elements, even though partially differentiated by context, should be more similar to each other than to other elements. While repeated elements in a sequence do not destroy the sequencing, they should constitute weak links in the associational chain. In structural models such as Lashley's, however, there should be no particular problem deciding which movement should follow the repeated one, for there are no event-to-event associations.

Wickelgren (1966) investigated the issue of repetition in short-term memory for lists of nine letters. In some lists, a letter was repeated twice and followed by a different letter in each case. During recall when an error was made on an item

---

[4] It may be noted that this explanation partially answers the problem mentioned earlier that the same movement varies with context. According to Wickelgren, movements that are conceptually the same may actually be represented differently if they occur in different contexts.

```
1 4 3 6 4 5 4 2 . . .        Normal sequence
1 4 3 6 4 5 4 3 . . .        Out-of-order associated event
                _
1 4 3 6 4 5 4 6 . . .        Out-of-order unassociated event
                _
1 4 3 6 4 5 3 . . .          Out-of-order control (doesn't follow
              _                  repeated event)
```

Figure 5 Examples of different types of out-of-order events in the repeated event experiment.

following a repeated item that error was often an intrusion of the item that followed the repeated one at the other place in the list. Such associative intrusions were more common than in control lists without repeated elements. These results are consistent with an event-to-event associative model.

Short-term memory may be rather different than well learned skills, however, so we explored the repeated elements problem in our skills paradigm.[5] Six lights and six response keys were used instead of eight as in the earlier experiment. In this case, however, one of the lights occurred three places in a sequence, each time followed by a different light, so the total event sequence was eight in length. As before, the sequence recycled after the last item. The order of lights was different for each of 12 subjects, but all sequences obeyed the same structure. An example of one sequence is 14364542. . . . Each subject practiced on the fixed sequence over 400 cycles in one session. During the second session, when all subjects were quite proficient on the task, 30% of the lights were out of order and the remaining lights occurred as expected in the learned sequence.

Of particular interest are the reaction times and errors to the out of sequence lights, and they were classified into three types as illustrated in Figure 5. On some occasions the repeated light occurred in its proper order but was followed by an out-of-order light. If the out-of-order light normally followed the repeated event at another place in the sequence it was called an associated light. Thus, for the illustrative sequence, if 14364 is followed by 3 or by 2, then 3 and 2 are associated events. If a repeated light is followed by one that normally does not follow the repetition in any position (lights 1 and 6 in the illustration sequence), it was called an unassociated event. Finally, any out-of-order light following a nonrepeated light is a control. If Wickelgren's (1969) associative hypothesis is correct, out-of-order but associated lights should result in faster reaction times and fewer errors than either unassociated or control lights, since occurrence of the repeated light should elicit all of its associates.

The reaction times and proportion of errors to the three types of out-of-order events are shown in Table I. The results conform to expectations, but statistically not all of them are significant. The associated events were faster than

---

[5] This experiment is not published elsewhere.

Table I
Mean Reaction Times (msec) and Proportion of
Errors for Out-of-Order Events

	Associated	Unassociated	Control
RT	506	516	532
Error	0.095	0.112	0.144

control events for all 12 subjects ($p < .01$) and more accurate for 9 subjects, with 2 ties and 1 reversal ($p < .05$). Although 8 of 12 subjects show faster reaction times and greater accuracy for associated than for unassociated events, these two comparisons are not significant. Examination of the table shows, however, that unassociated events are faster and less error prone than control events. Why would that be since both are controls in the sense that neither is associated with a repeated event? One possibility is that events following the repeated one are relatively ambiguous and hence are not strongly prepared for. In the absence of a strong expectation, any out-of-sequence event following a repeated light tends to be responded to faster than out-of-sequence events following nonrepeated lights, although associated events are responded to fastest of all. This tentative explanation is consistent with the Wickelgren hypothesis that repeated elements produce weak links in the associative chain.

To check the explanation, the data were analyzed from the first session in which the subjects responded as rapidly as they could to lights that always occurred in their proper order. If the linkage between a repeated event and ensuing events is rather weak, because of associative ambiguity, those events should be responded to rather slowly or with high errors. The relevant data are shown in Table II. Although reaction times do not differ among event types, errors do differ. As predicted, 9 of 12 subjects exhibited higher error rates for events following repeated events than for controls ($p < .05$). When these data are put together with the earlier data there is sufficient consistency to conclude that a repeated event elicits associations of all the events that follow it in different positions.

This second experiment using a somewhat different method supports the conclusion of the first experiment that some skills are represented in memory as associations between successive movements or events. The particular skills studied in the two experiments are of a particular type, however. They have no inherent structure other than linear ordering of events. Thus, we have mainly shown that for unstructured sequences of eight or nine events a position representation is not adopted and instead event-to-event associations are formed. This outcome might have been expected from general memory theory and observations of absolute judgments (Keele, 1973; Miller, 1956). When the number of events exceed about half a dozen there are too many for strict position recall, since that involves only one level or one dimension of organiza-

Table II

Mean Reaction time (msec) and Average Number
of Errors per Subject to Different Event Types

	Next event following repeated event	Repeated events	Control events
RT	267	265	270
Errors	3.45	2.83	1.33

tion. Instead they are recalled in a highly structured manner. If the events are quite unrelated to one another, associations between successive events are likely to be used. But when some other basis exists for categorizing events, recall is structured around categories or in a hierarchical organization (e.g., Mandler, 1967; Nelson and Smith, 1972). The issue arises, therefore, whether movement sequences with a possible structural basis other than linear positions lead to storage modes other than event-to-event associations.

B. Higher Order Structures

The issue of higher order structure in skills was investigated by Restle and Burnside (1972) using a procedure very similar to our own. Six buttons were placed beneath a six-light display. Lights came on every 0.7 sec and subjects tried to execute the corresponding button responses coincident with light onsets. Responses preceding or following the light by 0.3 sec were defined as correct and others were errors. In this paradigm the data of major interest are errors, whereas in our experiments reaction time was of major interest. Points of transition from correct responses to errors should given hints about the structure in memory.

In one study by Restle and Burnside, sequences of 16 lights were used. An example is 1234666662323543. After the last light the sequence recycled with no break. This sequence is composed of a run (1234), a reverse run (543), repetitions (66666), and a trill (232). Subjects watched the pattern of lights until they felt they had learned it and then began responding. The issue, of course, is whether the structure influences performance.

High error rates were produced to the last 6 in the repetitions (the error was often 2, anticipation of the next subsequence), to the first 2 in the trill (the error was often 6, a repetition overrun), and to the 5 in the reverse run. Following the first run of 1234, a common error was to make response 5. Quite clearly, therefore, subjects used the organization inherent in the list for structuring their own performance. If the beginning part of the sequence is a run, subjects apparently apply the rule, "generate a run beginning with 1." When the stopping point is forgotten, 5 is a likely error despite the fact that in the actual sequence it never follows 4 and hence should have no associative basis. Errors in general tend to occur at the beginning and end of units as though subjects had encoded a rule but forgot the termination point of one unit and the starting point of the next.

This first experiment by Restle and Burnside involved structured units but no higher level structure that relates units. In a second study they compared the sequence 123234345456654543432321 with the sequence 43245612365423 4321345543. The subunits of three elements are identical in the two cases but in the former case the units are also organized at a second level. Those people learning the more organized sequence made fewer errors in total, and they particularly made fewer errors at the transition between runs. As in studies of verbal memory, hierarchical structure appears to facilitate the learning process.

Lashley's conjecture that the representation of skills consists of structures into which events are placed appears, therefore, to be correct when movement sequences have permissible structures. When higher order rules or structures are present, they take precedence and override a mechanism based on sequential associations. In Restle's terminology a particular structure might be specified as: $M[T(R[T])]$ where M refers to mirror image, T refers to transposition, and R to repeat. Successive sets of parentheses denote successive levels in a hierarchy, i.e., at the lowest level transpositions occur; at the next higher level repeats occur; and so on. This particular structure stands apart from particular event assignments, as Lashley suggested. When the number of ordered events and the beginning elements are known, the rest of the events can be rule generated. Thus, if 6 lights are used, as in the Restle and Burnside study, and the first light is 1, then the rule application results in 1212232365655454. 1 is transposed to 2, the 2-element unit is repeated, the 4-element unit is transposed, and the 8-element unit is mirrored.

The conclusions regarding serial ordering of skills is very similar to conclusions regarding ordered memory for verbal materials. Serial lists of words apparently can consist in part of associations between successive events. Thus, some studies (e.g., Breckenridge and Dixon, 1970) found positive transfer from serial learning to paired associate learning when the pairs were constructed from successive words of the serial list. On the other hand, when more complex structures are available, people appear to use those rather than sequential association (Estes, 1972).

In everyday skills, event-to-event structures and higher order structures probably both exist. Many movement sequences have little or no repetition of elements and the elements are not spatially or otherwise related to each other except by direct association. The pattern of foot and hand movements in shifting an automobile may be such an example. On the other hand, musical skills almost certainly involve higher order rules. Even among lower animals, some skills may be rule governed rather than consisting solely of sequential associations. Fentress (1973b), in observing grooming patterns of mice, noted that the same component movement appeared in different grooming units. Nevertheless, the response to follow the repeated component was quite predictable by knowledge of the grooming unit in which the repetition was embedded. As seen earlier, an associative theory akin to Wickelgren's (1969) can handle the problem of repeated elements. Fentress noted in addition, however, that the unpredictability of a mouse's response was much greater near the beginning and end of units. This is reminiscent of Restle's observations, suggesting organization by units rather than strict sequential associations.

C. The Integration of Timing with Motor Programs

Almost all skills are finely timed as well as ordered. If a movement occurs in the correct order, but grossly out of time, the skill may completely fail. How is the timing integrated with the sequencing? The sequence representation and timing might be independent so that one program specifies sequencing and another attaches timing parameters as the sequence is unfolded. If so, then the same sequence could be readily executed with different time constraints. Alternatively, sequencing and timing might be integrated and inseparable.

Glencross (1973) observed handle cranking and noted that although different people cranked at different speeds, the relative time of different component movements remained rather constant. The duration of each component divided by the total cycle time was about the same for different people. Armstrong (1970) taught people patterns of lever movements. During reproduction from memory, relative timing of the different components of the pattern remained approximately constant although total time for the pattern varied. These results suggest that while overall speed is a parameter that can be attached to a motor program, the relative timing is part of the program itself. However, neither Glencross nor Armstrong instructed people to use different timing. Furthermore, the timing on those tasks may have been highly determined by mechanical constraints of the apparatus and limbs. A task is needed in which time constraints are arbitrarily imposed during training. Once the skill is well established, conditions are established in which the timing is no longer advantageous. In such a case does the learned timing persist?

Summers (1974) trained people to press the corresponding nine response keys to a repeating nine-light pattern. The sequence was different for each person, but an example is 591742683 and so on, repetitively. During a first session, subjects learned the sequence with no attempt to learn timing, but during the second session they were informed of the timing and attempted to learn it. For one group (551), the interval between one response and the next light was either 500 or 100 msec in the following rhythm: 500-500-100-500-500-100-

500-500-100 and so on.[6] Thus, the 9-element event pattern is matched with a 9-element time pattern. Another group (511) had similar training except the time pattern involved a long pause and two shorts (500-100-100). There were also two control groups. One had a constant 300 msec interval between one response and the next signal. The other had randomly determined intervals of 100, 300, and 500 msec that changed on each run through the sequence.

By the end of the second session, subjects were able to both reproduce the event sequence and the time pattern even when the lights were turned off and the pattern had to be reproduced entirely from memory. The time patterns as produced from memory at the end of training are shown in Figure 6. Of interest later is that the short and long interresponse time, when reproduction is from memory, are in about a 2:1 ratio.

During the third session the instructions were changed. Subjects were told to respond as rapidly as possible while keeping errors to a minimum; timing was no longer important. The critical question is whether subjects can discard the slow portions of the timing pattern they were trained on in order to produce all elements of the sequence as rapidly as possible. The results are shown in Figure 7.

All groups do respond faster than previously, but the two groups trained with time patterns are still influenced by the pattern of training, particularly group 511. For that group the time structure remains slow-fast-fast, although the exact proportions are changed somewhat from training. The 551 group, though retaining some time structure, has departed from the slow-slow-fast structure of training to slow-medium-fast under speeded conditions. Moreover, when the data are analyzed separately for the first block and last block of 10 blocks of speed trials, the 511 group exhibits virtually no change in the time structure. The 551 group, however, changes from a clear time structure on the first block to a near flat function on the tenth block.

Apparently, in some instances, timing is an integral part of a motor program and cannot be entered independently of the sequencing. This is apparently true only for some time patterns, however; for other patterns the trained timing rapidly deteriorates.

D. Rhythm and Timing

Some insight into why the 511 group differed from the 551 group might be gathered from a consideration of rhythm. Earlier we concluded that unpatterned sequences of events are stored as event-to-event associations. However, when

---

[6] The response to stimulus intervals in Summer's study were 500 or 100 msec. When a normal reaction time to the stimuli is added to these response-stimulus intervals, the total response to response intervals are closer to 2:1 ratio than 5:1. This is important for a later discussion about rhythmicity.

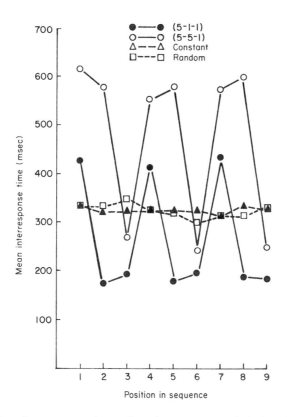

Figure 6 Mean interresponse times when the sequence and timing of responses are reproduced from memory.

events are organized into structures such as hierarchies, the sequence is much easier to learn and event-to-event associations are overridden. A similar issue arises for timing: Are some time patterns structurally simpler than others and hence easier to learn and more durable than others?

One structural basis for timing is rhythm. Martin (1972) suggests that rhythms are symmetrical, hierarchical structures of time patterns in which all the elements in the output occur at equal time intervals. Because it is hierarchical, the number of elements in a pattern must be a power of 2 if the hierarchical tree involves only binary branching. Martin only discusses binary branching, but rhythms could be based on more complex groupings such as powers of 3 (tertiary branching) or combinations with tertiary grouping at one level and binary branching at another. Groupings based on even larger elements such as 5 or 7 may be possible in principle but difficult for people to perceive or produce in practice. The implication of this hierarchical notion is that if the number of events in a sequence is neither a power nor a multiple of 2 or 3, then blank elements must be inserted at appropriate points to make it appear rhythmic. For example, if there are 5 events in a repeating pattern, the sequence may not appear rhythmic unless 1, 3, or 4 blank time intervals are inserted to bring the number of elements including blanks to 6 (multiple of 3), to 8 (a power of 2), or 9 (a power of 3). Each element, including the blanks, would then occur at equal time intervals.

Now consider the 511 sequence used in Summers' experiment. Recall that when subjects produced the timing from memory, the ratio of slow to fast interresponse intervals was about 2:1. Furthermore, to be rhythmic each sub-element of a sequence must fall at equal time intervals. The subsequence slow-fast-fast could then be viewed as a sequence of four elements: the slow interval is composed of two elements equal in length to each fast element. One subelement is identified with a sequence event and one is blank or a null event. For example, one portion of the sequence 591742683 ... in that experiment would become 5-blank-9-1, with each of the four resulting elements appearing at equal time intervals. Because the number of elements is 4, a power of 2, it is rhythmic.

The 551 timing in contrast is difficult to make rhythmic. If each slow element is composed of two subelements equal in length to the fast elements, producing,

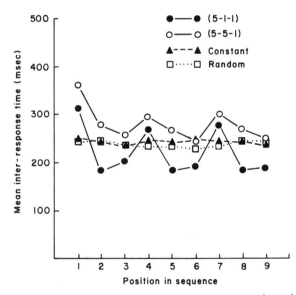

Figure 7 Mean interresponse time when people attempt to produce the sequence as rapidly as possible without regard to timing.

for example, the subsequence 5-blank-9-blank-1, then there are a total of five elements which is neither a power nor a multiple of 2 or 3. If subjects attempt to make the slow elements three times as slow as the fast elements, producing 5-blank-blank-9-blank-blank-1, the result is still a poor rhythm.

Thus, the reason that the 551 timing may not persist as an integral part of the motor program is that structurally it is more awkward than the 511 timing.

This analysis of Summer's experiment is obviously *post hoc*. Unfortunately there appear to be few, if any, studies examining rhythm from a motor skills standpoint. A study that illustrates the role of rhythm in perception and immediate memory, however, was conducted by Sturges and Martin (1974). They presented either 7- or 8-item sequences of high and low tones at equal intervals per tone and at either 3.3/sec or 4.4/sec. Each sequence was either repeated, for a total of 14 or 16 equal interval tones, or a slightly different sequence was repeated, and subjects judged whether the sequences were the same or different. The 7-item sequences were constructed by deleting the last item from an 8-item sequence. From the earlier discussion it may be recalled that to be apparently rhythmic, a sequence must contain a number of elements that is a power or multiple of 2 or 3. Therefore, some of the 8-item sequences were rhythmic,[7] but none of the 7-item sequences could be, at least by simple criteria of rhythmicity. The results demonstrated the rhythmic 8-item sequences to be judged more accurately than the shorter 7-item sequences. Furthermore, within 8-item sequences, rhythmic ones were judged more accurately than nonrhythmic ones.

Although the evidence is not as clear as it is for event structures, it appears that rhythmic time structures influence skills differently than arbitrary time patterns. When the timing is rhythmic, it may well be learned more easily, and it appears to become an integral part of the movement sequence and not easily divorced from the sequencing. Although the tempo can be altered, rhythm cannot. When the time structure is more arbitrary, on the other hand, it appears to have a more transient relationship with the sequencing, and it gradually becomes altered to a simpler structure such as constant time intervals.

IV. Summary

A major aspect of motor skills is the sequencing of movements, and this chapter is primarily concerned with the memorial representation of sequencing. An S-R chaining theory of sequence representation is inadequate to explain the

---

[7] In the Sturges and Martin study, the first and fifth items of rhythmic 8-item sequences were accented. In the nonrhythmic sequences, the accent fell on the first and fourth or first and sixth elements. Details of rhythm rules can be found in Martin (1972).

rich complexity of skilled performance. Some skills can be performed in the absence of kinesthetic feedback, suggesting a central representation. Even when feedback is intimately involved in movement, its role appears to be more of a monitor for detection and correction of errors than for stimulating subsequent movements. Many skills, therefore, appear represented in the central memory structure as a motor program, rather than as a peripheral-central S-R chain. This conception of skill, simple as it is, when combined with conceptions of the role of feedback, has potential implications for skill training.

The central representation (motor program) could be a chain of associations, though not involving peripheral feedback as stimuli. Although this representation appears to underlie movement sequences unstructured except for linear ordering of events, sequences with inherent structure appear to be stored as hierarchical structures or movement generating rules. The timing of events rather than being independent of sequencing appears to be an integral part of the motor program, particularly for rhythmic time structures.

Acknowledgments

Work in this chapter occurred while supported by an Office of Naval Research Contract No. N00014-67-A-0446-004 and by the Advanced Research Projects Agency of the Department of Defense and was monitored by the Air Force Office of Scientific Research under Contract No. F44620-73-C-0056; their support is gratefully acknowledged. We would like to thank Scott Kelso, Beth Kerr, Ray Klein, and Mary Jo Nissen for their helpful comments.

References

Adams, J.A. (1971). *J. Mot. Behav.* **3**, 111–150.
Armstrong, T.R. (1970). "Training for the Production of Memorized Movement Patterns" *Tech. Rep.* No. 26. Human Performance Center, Univ. of Michigan, Ann Arbor, Michigan.
Bizzi, E. (1974). *Sci. Amer.* **231**, 100–106.
Bossom, J. (1974). *Brain Res.* **71**, 285–296.
Bossom, J., and Ommaya, A.K. (1968). *Brain* **91**, 161–172.
Breckenridge, R.L., and Dixon, T.R. (1970). *J. Exp. Psychol.* **83**, 126–130.
Brumbach, W.B. (1969). *Nat. Coll. Phys. Educ. Ass. Proc.* **pp.** 36–40.
Docherty, D. (1973). Doctoral Dissertaion, University of Oregon Eugene (unpublished).
Estes, W.K. (1972). *In* "Coding Processes in Human Memory" (A.W. Melton and E. Martin, eds.), p. 161. Winston, Washington, D.C.
Evarts, E.V., and Ranji, J. (1974). *Brain Res.* **71**, 479–494.
Fentress, J.C. (1973a). *Science* **179**, 704–705.
Fentress, J.C. (1973b). *Nature (London)* **244**, 52–53.
Glencross, D.J. (1973). *Ergonomics* **16**, 765–776.
Glencross, D.J. (1975). *Psychol. Bull.* (in press).
Greenwald, A.G. (1970). *Psychol. Rev.* **77**, 73–99.

Hinde, R.A. (1969). *Quart. J. Exp. Psychol.* **21**, 106–126.

Howard, I.P., and Templeton, W.B. (1966). "Human Spatial Orientation." Wiley, New York.

Kalikow, D.N. (1974). "Information Processing Models and Computer Aids for Human Performance: Final Report Second Language Learning." Technical Report No. 2841. Bolt, Beranek & Newman, Cambridge, Massachusetts.

Kalikow, D.N., and Rollins, A.M. (1973). "Information Processing Models and Computer Aids for Human Performance: Technical Report Second Language Learning." Technical Report No. 2654. Bolt, Beranek & Newman, Cambridge, Massachusetts.

Keele, S.W. (1968). *Psychol. Bull.* **70**, 387–403.

Keele, S.W. (1973). "Attention and Human Performance." Goodyear, Pacific Palisades, California.

Keele, S.W. (1975). *In* "Attention and Performance V" (P.M.A. Rabbitt and S. Dornic, eds.), p. 357. Academic Press, New York.

Kelso, J.A.S., Stelmach, G.E., and Wanamaker, W.M. (1974). *J. Mot. Behav.* **6**, 179–190.

Konishi, M. (1965). *Z. Tierpsychol.* **22**, 770–783.

Lashley, K.S. (1951). *In* "Cerebral Mechanisms in Behavior" (L.A. Jeffress, ed.). Wiley, New York.

Lawther, J.D. (1968). "The Learning of Physical Skills." Prentice-Hall, Englewood Cliffs, New Jersey.

Lazlo, J.I. (1966). *Quart. J. Exp. Psychol.* **18**, 1–8.

Lazlo, J.I. (1967). *Quart. J. Exp. Psychol.* **19**, 344–349.

MacNeilage, P.F. (1970). *Psychol. Rev.* **77**, 182–196.

Mandler, G. (1967). *In* "The Psychology of Learning and Motivation" (K.W. Spence and J.T. Spence, eds.), Vol. I, p. 328. Academic Press, New York.

Marsden, C.D., Merton, P.A., and Morton, H.B. (1972). *Nature (London)* **238**, 140–143.

Martin, J.G. (1972). *Psychol. Rev.* **79**, 487–509.

Matthews, P.B.C. (1964). *Physiol. Rev.* **44**, 219–288.

Merton, P.A. (1972). *Sci. Amer.* **226**, 30–37.

Miller, G.A. (1956). *Psychol. Rev.* **63**, 81–97.

Mott, F.W., and Sherrington, C.S. (1895). *Proc. Roy. Soc. London* **57**, 481–488.

Nelson, T.O., and Smith, E.E. (1972). *J. Exp. Psychol.* **95**, 388–396.

Nickerson, R.S., and Stevens, K.N. (1973). *IEEE Trans. Audio Electroacoustics* **21**, 445–455.

Nottebohm, F. (1970). *Science* **167**, 950–956.

Pew, R.W. (1966). *J. Exp. Psychol.* **71**, 764–771.

Pew, R.W. (1974). *In* "Human Information Processing: Tutorials in Performance and Cognition" (B.H. Kantowitz, ed.), p. 1. Erlbaum, New York.

Phillips, C.G. (1969). *Proc. Roy. Soc., Ser. B* **173**, 141–174.

Pronko, N.H. (1969). *Psychol. Today* **2**, 52.

Restle, F., and Burnside, B.L. (1972). *J. Exp. Psychol.* **95**, 299–307.

Schmidt, R.A. (1975). *Psychol. Rev.* **82**, 225–260.

Smith, J.L., Roberts, E.M., and Atkins, E. (1972). *Amer. J. Phys. Med.* **51**, 225–238.

Stelmach, G.E., Kelso, J.A.S., Wallace, S.A., and Clark, J.E. (1975). *J. Exp. Psychol.* (in press).

Sturges, P.T., and Martin, J.G. (1974). *J.Exp. Psychol.* **102**, 377–383.

Summers, J.J. (1973). Master's Thesis, University of Oregon, Eugene (unpublished).

Summers, J.J. (1974). Doctoral Dissertation, University of Oregon, Eugene (unpublished).

Sussman, H.M. (1972). *Psychol. Bull.* **77**, 262–272.

Taub, E., and Berman, A.J. (1968). *In* "The Neuropsychology of Spatially Oriented Behavior" (S.J. Freedman, ed.), p. 173. Dorsey, Homewood, Illinois.

Taub, E., Perrella, P., and Barro, G. (1973). *Science* **181**, 959–960.
Taylor, A., and Cody, F.W.J. (1974). *Brain Res.* **71**, 523–530.
Vallbo, A.B. (1971). *J. Physiol. (London)* **218**, 405–431.
Wickelgren, W.A. (1966). *J. Exp. Psychol.* **72**, 853–858.
Wickelgren, W.A. (1969). *Psychol. Bull.* **76**, 1–15.
Wilson, D.M. (1961). *J. Exp. Biol.* **38**, 471–490.

Attention and Movement

Raymond M. Klein

I. Introduction

In the late nineteenth century Hughlings Jackson proposed a hierarchical view of motor control (See Phillips, 1973). At the lowest level he placed a reflexive control system with very direct sensory-motor connections. At the middle level, the connections are less direct, and somewhat more flexible. At the highest level is an integrative, executive control system which is responsible for the coordination of the lower levels to produce the finely controlled movements characteristic of voluntary behavior. Since Jackson's early proposal technological advances (in stimulation, recording, staining, microscopy, etc.) and physiological and anatomical findings have greatly improved our understanding of the control of movement by spinal mechanisms (Jackson's lower level) and by the motor cortex and cerebellum (Jackson's middle level). Unfortunately, there has been little progress in our understanding of the control of movement by the highest level in Jackson's hierarchy.[1]

It is my view that our understanding of the voluntary control of movement will benefit greatly from a psychological framework that distinguishes conscious from unconscious mental activity. This distinction can be incorporated within an information-processing framework. Many studies of human performance during perceptual tasks have revealed a bottleneck in the processing sequence. This bottleneck, often referred to as attention, is closely related to conscious awareness (Posner and Klein, 1973) in the sense that the processing operations which occupy it are conscious while those which do not are unconscious. This attentional mechanism may also perform the integrative, executive functions characteristic of the voluntary control of movement (MacKay, 1966).

The main purpose of this chapter will be to illustrate how the concept of attention can be used and has been applied to problems in the perception and production of movement. I will begin with a brief history of the concept of attention and an outline of the particular view of the concept which I have adopted. I will then discuss the role of attentional biases in the pervasive phenomenon of visual dominance and I will examine the attentional requirements of motor control. Some sections will concentrate on findings, while others will emphasize methodological issues or suggestions for future research.

II. Attention

A. Historical Survey

What is attention?

> Everyone knows what attention is. It is the taking possession by the mind, in clear and vivid form of one out of what seem several simultaneous possible objects or trains of thought. . . . It implies withdrawal from some things in order to deal effectively with others [James, 1890, p. 403].

At the turn of the century this view of conscious attention was at the very core of experimental psychology (Titchener, 1908). An overreliance on subjective reports and inadequate methods and tools of measurement led to the rise of

---

[1] Advances in microelectrode techniques have enabled investigators to record central nervous system activity during voluntary movement in alert and freely behaving preparations. When combined with appropriate behavioral manipulations this technique promises to tell us a great deal about the control of the lower levels by volition (see, e.g., Evarts and Tanji, 1974; Fetz and Finicchio, 1971).

behaviorism and the subsequent (but transitory) decline of the study of attention and other mental events.

During World War II practical considerations led to the study of human performance on watchkeeping (vigilance) tasks. The immediate aim of these studies was to understand the performance decrement that occurred during long radar watches. The concept of attention resurfaced when it was found useful for explaining vigilance performance as a function of variables such as time on task, perceptual load, and environmental stressors. Interest in attention was further stimulated when the brain stem reticular formation was implicated in the sleep-wakefulness cycle (Moruzzi and Magoun, 1949) and the notion of a brain mechanism related to awareness became an acceptable idea. Perhaps the most significant factor in the return of "attention" to the forefront of psychology was the development of computers and communication theory. These developments led to a new *Zeitgeist* in which man is viewed as an information-processing system. This view provides a framework for the objective study of mental processes which are "hidden" from direct observation. In particular, by viewing attention as a selective filter or a limited capacity mechanism psychologists gave the concept the operational validity that it did not possess in the early days of psychology.

This information processing viewpoint has led to an effort to identify and describe information-processing stages which intervene between stimulus and response. For example, stimulus identification, memory retrieval, response selection, response initiation, and response execution stages have been assumed to follow the presentation of a stimulus. Theories of human performance are concerned with the attentional requirements of these processing stages. Two views of attention have dominated the human performance literature. One view assumes that there is a bottleneck at a specific location within the information-processing sequence. The second assumes that there is a limited capacity system that can be flexibly allocated to different stages or types of processing.

The view of attention as a bottleneck in the information-processing sequence has its origins in the classic work of Broadbent (1958). He placed the bottleneck early in the sequence, prior to the memory retrieval stage. Since the evidence for this assumption is rather detailed, I have chosen an illustrative example. Suppose you are wearing headphones and a different message is presented to each ear. You are asked to repeat each word as it is presented to one ear while ignoring the other message. Such a task is called dichotic shadowing. When shadowing a message to one ear, one is completely unaware of the semantic content of the unattended message. If the speaker changes languages (e.g., English to French) this is usually not noticed. There is usually no memory for the unattended material. When you are asked to respond whenever you hear a certain word (in either ear) you rarely miss the word when it is presented to the attended ear, but you miss it most of the time when it is presented to the unattended ear. On the other hand, physical characteristics of the unattended message are processed. If the voice switches from male to female, for instance, this usually is noticed. These results strongly suggested that attending to the message to one ear involves filtering out the other message, so that it is not processed beyond the level of its physical characteristics. This view meshed nicely with physiological data supporting the notion of peripheral filters mediating attention (Hernandes-Peon *et al.*, 1956).

This view was challenged by some (e.g., Deutsch and Deutsch, 1963; Norman, 1968), and subsequent studies demonstrate that the bottleneck is not necessarily located early in the processing sequence. Careful experiments reveal that the original physiological evidence for peripheral filtering was hopelessly flawed (see Milner, 1970, pp. 282–287). Several studies of shadowing demonstrate that the meaning of nonattended words is activated. When the unattended word is a synonym of the attended word, reaction time (RT) to shadow the attended word is greater than when the two words are unrelated (Lewis, 1970). MacKay (1973) found that unattended words influence the interpretation which is given to an attended ambiguous sentence. These studies, and others (Corteen and Wood, 1972; Posner and Boies, 1971) demonstrate that memory retrieval may be automatic in the sense that it does not require attention.

One proposal for dealing with these findings has been to place the bottleneck later in the sequence, in the initiation of responses (Keele, 1973) or in the competition for response processes (Milner, 1970; Shallice, 1972). Milner, for example, suggests that,

> ... perhaps more progress would be made if investigators were to abandon the idea that selection or filtering is carried out in the sensory pathways and were to entertain instead the hypothesis that the process is a consequence of competition among central processes for control of the motor system which can deal with only one response sequence at a time [Milner, 1970, p. 260].

Evidence discussed below (see Section IV,B), however, shows that in certain situations responses may be initiated without the involvement of attention. Furthermore, as the tip-of-the-tongue phenomenon amply demonstrates, memory retrieval may require a great deal of conscious attention. Thus it seems that attention cannot be tied down to a specific location within the information processing sequence.

An alternative view (Kahneman, 1973; Laberge, 1975; Moray, 1967; Posner and Synder, 1975b) proposes that attention can be allocated flexibly to different information processing stages. This is the type of theory I have adopted and will describe below. My views are based largely on studies of attention during perceptual tasks and have been influenced by Posner (Posner and Boies, 1971; Posner and Klein, 1973; Posner and Snyder, 1974a,b), as well as Keele (1973), Kahneman (1973), and Shallice (1972).

B. A View of Attention

I view attention as a brain mechanism of limited capacity. Attention can be allocated to different sensory inputs, mental operations, memory locations, response processes, etc. Because attention is limited in capacity its commitment to one task reduces the likelihood that nonattended tasks will have access to attention. Thus interference will occur whenever two simultaneous operations require attention.[2] This fact suggests that interference techniques may be useful for measuring the attention demands of mental activities (perceptual, as well as motor). These techniques will be discussed in Section II,C.

When will a task require attention? What functions does this mechanism perform? These are empirical questions. Many operations can be performed automatically, that is, without attention. For example, a visually presented word automatically activates habitual associations such as the name of the word and semantic associates. On the other hand, many nonhabitual operations require attention (Posner and Snyder, 1975a). The retrieval of the meaning of unfamiliar words, for example, may require a conscious search of memory. The allocation of attention to one input source does not seem to affect the accumulation of information about simultaneous unattended items, although it does reduce the likelihood that unattended items will interrupt the attended task. The consequences of attending one input source are that the attended items will be remembered and responded to, while unattended items will not. Thus, attention serves the important function of selecting the stimuli, mental operations, and memory codes that control our present and future responses. I believe this brain mechanism also performs the integrative, executive functions which Jackson placed at the highest level in his hierarchy of motor control.

A tentative and oversimplified diagram illustrating this view of attention is shown in Figure 1. Evidence for this model can be found in the studies cited at the end of Section II,A. Although some of the material in this chapter is consistent with this model (and may have been influential in my adoption of it) the reader should be aware that I am not presenting this material to validate the model. My goal is to explore the contributions which such a model can make to the study of movement.

C. Measuring Attention Demands:
The Secondary Task Technique

The limited-capacity nature of attention suggests a simple method for determining the attentional requirements of a particular task or task component. The

---

[2] It should be pointed out that all limited capacity theories of attention do not entail this prediction. Kahneman (1973), for example, views attention as a pool of capacity. Two tasks requiring attention will interfere in his model only when the amount of capacity demanded exceeds the amount supplied. I view attention as a discrete mechanism. When this mechanism is occupied by a task, any new signals will have difficulty gaining access to attention.

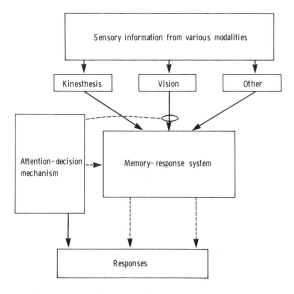

Figure 1 A view of attention. There are four basic structural components: (1) Sensory modalities which convey information from receptors to the memory-response system; (2) a memory-response system which contains sensory, abstract and response related representations that mediate perception and action; (3) effector mechanisms which are activated to produce responses to changes in internal and external conditions; (4) an attention-decision mechanism which is required for performing certain nonhabitual mental operations including the coordination of effector mechanisms. Several assumptions mentioned in the text are stated more formally below: (a) the attention decision mechanism is limited in capacity. Simultaneous tasks which require attention will necessarily interfere with each other. (b) Attention can be allocated flexibly to different processing stages, locations in memory, mental operations, effector mechanisms, etc. (attention is allocated to the visual modality in the figure). (c) The commitment of attention increases the likelihood that attended items will be remembered and responded to. It reduces the likelihood that the attended task will be interrupted. (d) The automatic activation of representations in the memory-response system by sensory inputs depends upon compatibility and previous experience, and is not affected by attention.

method is simply to measure the amount of interference when a simultaneous secondary task is performed. This method was actually suggested as early as 1886 by the French physiologist Jacques Loeb. He showed that the maximum pressure which the flexor muscles of the hand can exert upon a dynamometer decreases when the subject attempts to do mental work. His student, Jeanette Welch (1898), calculated a constant of attention for various tasks such as visual monitoring, adding, and reading by comparing the maximum pressure exerted during these activities with that exerted during no mental work. In recent years the measurement of processing demands during perceptual tasks has burgeoned. The interested reader is directed to excellent reviews by Kerr (1973) and Kahneman (1973, Chapter 10).

Interference between two tasks is not always based upon attentional limitations. The difficulty we have talking while we eat is primarily due to the incompatible movements of the mouth and tongue which these activities entail. This type of interference is referred to as structural (Kahneman, 1973) and the example I have given is, I admit, extreme. Structural interference refers to a limitation within a specific perceptual, memory, or response system. Because it is rather easy for structural interference to masquerade as an attentional limitation, attempts should be made to minimize it when choosing a secondary task.

Many investigators have used the secondary task to probe the attentional requirements of the primary task. When this method is used the experimenter should examine primary task performance in the absence of the secondary task. When the probe (secondary) task affects the primary task performance it cannot be used as a pure measure of the demands of the primary task. Data should also be collected on the probe task alone. The experimenter should perform a subtraction (e.g., probe RT during primary task − probe RT alone) which will reflect the attention demands of the primary task.

III. Perception of Movement

A. Sources of Feedback

Evarts (1971) has discussed three categories of feedback that may be used in motor control: (1) the traditional sensory feedback from the movement itself, (2) knowledge of the motor commands or corollary discharge, and (3) knowledge of results. Feedback from a movement may be used at many levels. For example, information conveyed by spindle and tendon afferents about the state of a muscle may influence motor control monosynaptically and polysynaptically at the spinal level, or through relatively short loops through the cerebellum and motor cortex. This feedback may be directed at the same muscle, antagonists or synergists; its effect may be inhibitory or facilitory. Since we are interested in the conscious control of movement I will begin by discussing the extent to which these three categories of feedback have access to conscious attention.

Suppose you watch your hand as it traces a pattern. Direct information about the movement pattern will be conveyed by visual and kinesthetic pathways. There would be little disagreement that visual information has access to awareness. With kinesthesis, the situation is less clear-cut. The various sources of kinesthetic feedback (the receptors in the skin, joints and muscles) transmit different types of information concerning movement. In recent years it has generally been assumed that some of these sources do not have access to attention.

It is universally agreed that joint receptors provide information about limb position which can be used in conscious judgments. When the joint capsule is anesthetized, sensitivity to passive movement is reduced or absent (Goldscheider,

1889; Browne *et al.*, 1954; Provins, 1958). It is usually assumed that tactile feedback provides only crude information about movement (Howard and Templeton, 1966). For movements which do not involve contact with any external objects or other parts of the body, this view is probably correct, i.e., deformation of the skin near the moving joint is not likely to provide accurate feedback about position or movement. However, manual exploration of an object or the movements one makes when taking a shower can certainly be guided by tactile feedback. Furthermore, when force is exerted against an external object pressure signals from the skin may be very useful, while the joint receptors will tell nothing if no movement is produced.

In recent years it has generally been assumed that muscle receptors (spindle and tendon organs) provide information[3] which is used only subconsciously in motor control (Granit and Burke, 1973). Merton (1964, 1972) has been the most forceful proponent of this view that muscle is insentient. Merton points out that the information from spindles signals relative length (length relative to the contraction of the spindle produced by gamma activation) rather than absolute length. He uses the power-assisted steering analogy to suggest that the signals from these receptors could only confuse. Would a dial on the dashboard showing the state of the alignment detector be of any use to the driver? One counterargument (Howard and Templeton, 1966) is that the spindle discharge becomes perfectly decipherable when the amount of gamma innervation is known.

Merton cites good experimental and clinical evidence that the muscle spindles and tendon organs do not contribute to consciousness. Some investigators (Browne *et al.*, 1954; Gelfan and Carter, 1967; Provins, 1958) eliminated skin and joint information. They found complete insensitivity to passive movements. Bridley and Merton (1960) passively moved the eye by pulling on the insertion of the extraocular muscle. Although this muscle has spindles, the subject was unable to perceive any movement when vision was occluded. These results suggest that muscle receptors alone cannot subserve conscious judgments. Two recent studies, however, raise problems for this view.

Skavensky (1972) replicated the Brindley and Merton experiment on the sensitivity to passive eye movements in the dark. He used a more sensitive psychophysical procedure and a delicate suction contact lens arrangement to move the eye painlessly. It was found that highly practiced subjects could make judgments about the direction of passive eye movements, and could compensate

---

[3] Muscle spindles are embedded in the main muscle, and generally respond when stretched. The sensory portion of the spindle can be stretched either when the muscle in which it resides is stretched, or when the polar ends of the spindle are contracted by the action of gamma efferents. The Golgi tendon organs are found in the tendinous tissue which connects muscle to bone. These receptors respond to tension and changes in tension. See Matthews (1972) for a more detailed discussion.

for passively applied loads. Thus, spindle information may be used for judgments about eye movements. Goodwin *et al.* (1972) found that subjects consistently misperceived a vibration-induced movement of the arm. The vibratory stimulus probably disrupts feedback from muscle receptors but does not affect joint feedback. The illusion suggests that feedback from the muscle receptors can influence the conscious perception of movement. The conflict between these studies and those which suggest that muscle is insentient may soon be resolved. One might tentatively conclude that conscious judgments about limb movement may be influenced by spindle and tendon feedback and that experienced subjects may use spindle feedback for judgments about eye position and movement in the dark.

Knowledge about the motor commands issued to the muscles (efference) may play a role in the conscious perception of movement. This is suggested by the fact that it is possible to make relatively accurate active movements or force responses in the absence of sensory feedback (Lashley, 1917; Ommaya and Levine, summarized in Granit and Burke, 1973; Provins, 1958). It has even been suggested (Festinger *et al.*, 1967) that conscious experience is determined by efference.

In the performance literature "knowledge of results" usually refers to a form of augmented feedback about one's performance. For example, in a reaction time experiment the subject might be told the precise latency of his responses. Knowledge of results is not always augmented feedback, however, it may also be inherent in the task. For instance, in the absence of visual and kinesthetic feedback an attempt to bang a drum or place food in one's mouth will result in a unique sensory experience when the attempt is successful. This type of feedback can be carried over any sensory pathway. Although it will not always be sufficient to guide a movement knowledge of results is often used to monitor the success of one's actions (especially in musical skills and speech), and may mediate the learning of skills in the absence of other sources of feedback.

It appears that information from many sources can influence the perception of a movement. Some interesting questions may be raised concerning the limited capacity nature of attention. Are these sources normally coordinated in such a way that we have a unitary perception which is influenced by several modalities? Or is attention committed to one source at a time? For instance, when we watch our movements is our awareness of the kinesthetic or visual feedback, or both? This question has a long history. In 1899 Woodworth asked,

> If therefore, any sense may control a movement, we have to ask what the result will be when two senses are each in a position to do the work. . . . Will the movement obey two masters, or will it cleave to one and despise the other [Woodworth, 1899, p. 73].

Studies of conflict between vision and kinesthesis suggest that when these sources of feedback are both available attention is directed toward vision. For example, the following illusion was described at a recent conference on the control of movement and posture (Hagbarth, summarized in Granit and Burke, 1973): If a normal subject swings his arm in an arc around the elbow joint in a completely dark room and the arm is stroboscopically illuminated only when it is at $90°$, then the subject has the strong sensation that he is not really moving his arm at all. When the subject closes his eyes, the illusion disappears. This illusion is a most striking example of a phenomenon that has been called "visual dominance" or "visual capture." In the following sections I review studies which demonstrate the widespread occurrence of visual dominance and I will speculate on its origins.

B. Visual Dominance: Conflict

The term "visual capture" was first used by Tastevin (1937). His subjects viewed a plastic replica of one of their fingers protruding from under a cloth. The subject generally mistook the replica for his own finger which was concealed from view several centimeters away. Gibson (1943) independently demonstrated a similar effect. His subjects wore prism spectacles which made straight edges look curved. When the subjects watched themselves move their hand along an objectively straight edge their kinesthetic perception did not conflict with the visual perception: the edge was felt as curved. According to Gibson, "this dominance of vision over kinesthetic perception was so complete that when the subjects were instructed to dissociate the two, i.e. 'to feel it straight and see it curved' it was reported difficult or impossible to do so [p. 4]." Numerous experimental studies have confirmed these early demonstrations of visual dominance.

Rock and Victor (1964) had subjects examine a square object through a lens which made it appear rectangular. When later asked to select a matching object from a set using only touch, subjects who had examined the object with vision and touch concurrently chose a matching object that was almost identical to what they had seen. Visual dominance in judgments of size and shape has also been found by Kinney and Luria (1970) and Rock et al. (1965).

Visual-kinesthetic conflict has been most thoroughly studied in judgments of spatial location (e.g., Hay et al., 1965; Pick et al., 1969). In a typical experiment, the subject is wearing prism spectacles that displace the visual world about $10°-15°$. In the conflict conditions the subject looks at a finger of his outstretched hand and points to the felt or seen location of this finger (using his other hand, which is blocked from view). These conditions are compared to two nonconflict conditions (the subject points at the felt location of his finger without vision or at the seen location of a visual target) to assess the influence each modality has upon judgments of location within the other modality. One aspect of this procedure is an improvement over the Rock and Victor method: subjects are receiving the conflicting visual and kinesthetic information while the judgment is made. Thus, there is no reliance upon memory which may differ for the two modalities (e.g., see Posner, 1967). These studies (Hay et al., 1965; Pick et al., 1969) support the conclusions of Rock and Victor (1964): When the subject is presented with conflicting visual and kinesthetic feedback, his judgment of the felt position of his limb is dominated by the visual information.

Kinney and Luria (1970) studied visual-kinesthetic conflict in an underwater environment (visual targets are displaced because of the refraction that takes place as light passes from water to air at the subject's face mask). In one experiment, they trained blindfolded subjects to hit a bull's-eye with one hand while they were holding it in the other. After this task was learned to criterion, the subjects were allowed to look at the target before but not during their movement. This inaccurate visual information caused errors which indicated that the subjects were aiming at the displaced visual image. Thus, even a well-learned motor program acquired in the absence of vision is modified by conflicting visual input.

The studies discussed so far have been concerned with the immediate effect of conflict upon performance. There is another effect which occurs when we are allowed to view our moving hand in relation to nonmoving objects. If you look through displacing prisms which shift the visual field to the right, your initial attempts to grasp an object will be too far to the right. When this happens you will be aware of the discrepancy, and after a few more attempts the error is corrected (adaptation). When the prisms are removed, however, movements are too far to the left (aftereffect). Considerable evidence has been gathered by Harris (1965) for the view that the adjustment (adaptation and aftereffect) is mediated by a change in the felt position of the hand and arm rather than changes within the visual system or in visual-motor coordination. One example of the evidence cited by Harris is that adaptation is restricted to the exposed hand; it does not transfer to the unexposed hand. If the adjustment were within the visual system, for instance, the performance of the exposed and unexposed hands would be identical. The implication that the visual system is stable, while the kinesthetic system is extremely labile is consistent with the immediate effect of conflict on awareness and performance.

C. Visual Dominance: Natural Situations

The preceding demonstrations of visual dominance were obtained in relatively artificial situations, in which mirrors, lenses, an underwater environment, or mechanical deception were used to create a conflict between the two modalities. Visual dominance has also been demonstrated in more natural situations.

Walker (1972) observed that when subjects compare the lengths of two objects, one on their right and the other on their left, there is a tendency for the object on the left to be overestimated by vision, and underestimated by touch. He asked his subjects to make bilateral length comparisons while they examined objects by vision alone, touch alone (one object in each hand), or by both concurrently. When examining both concurrently, subjects were asked which felt longer or which looked longer. While the findings were not as striking as some of the more artificial demonstrations of visual dominance, they did reveal a natural tendency for subjects to use visual information when asked to make a kinesthetic judgment.

Visual dominance has also been demonstrated in a reaction time paradigm (Jordan, 1972; Klein and Posner, 1974, exp. III) which is quite different from those we have discussed so far. Jordan (1972) trained novice fencers to initiate a fencing move when a foil they were holding was deflected by a mechanical foil (thus giving rise to kinesthetic information). He measured RT to begin the movement in three different groups of subjects. The first group (kinesthetic) was blindfolded; the second (bimodal) was allowed to watch; and the third (visual) was also allowed to watch, but the mechanical foil was placed 15 cm from the subject's foil (in the other conditions the two foils were touching). This third group was intended as a visual control: The initial information was entirely visual. This condition is not purely visual, however, because the impact (about 80 msec after the mechanical foil begins to move) gives rise to kinesthetic information that is probably more intense than in the other conditions. As expected visual RT was slower than kinesthetic RT. More interesting, in the last test session RT in the bimodal condition was 27 msec slower than RT in the kinesthetic condition. A subsequent study by Klein and Posner (1974, exp. III) strengthens the generality of this finding. Their subjects made a two-choice response with their left hand to indicate the direction of a passive movement of their right forefinger. In one condition (bimodal) the movement was displayed on an oscilloscope as the finger was moved, while in another condition it was not (kinesthetic). Reaction time in the bimodal condition was 24 msec slower than in the kinesthetic condition. When two inputs signaling the same response occur simultaneously a statistical redundancy gain may be found: RT may be shorter than to either stimulus alone.[4] The finding that the response latency to a kinesthetic input is increased when simultaneous visual feedback is available suggests that kinesthetic feedback is not fully used in the presence of visual feedback.

D. Why Does Vision Dominate?

The occurrence of visual dominance is widespread. The view of attention adopted in this paper suggests a simple statement for summarizing the phenomenon: Vision has priority over kinesthesis for access to attention. This

---

[4] This will be found whenever (1) the subject uses both sources of information, and (2) the response latency distributions for the two inputs overlap (see Nickerson, 1973 for a discussion).

statement is descriptive, not explanatory. We are still left with the question: Why does vision have priority? Is visual dominance wired in and therefore a necessary consequence of the simultaneous presence of visual and kinesthetic information? Or does visual dominance result from a bias to attend vision when visual information appears sufficient for responding?

The developmental literature suggests that visual dominance may not be learned. In their review of perceptual integration in children Pick *et al.* (1967) found no evidence for developmental changes in visual dominance. In a spatial localization paradigm, Warren and Pick (1970) found no difference between second and sixth graders and adults in either visual dominance over kinesthesis, or the slight kinesthetic influence over vision. Since children who are 8 years old may already have had enough experience for dominance to become established, studies with infants would be more revealing. Two recent studies compared visual and kinesthetic control over certain infant behaviors. Lee and Aronson (1974) found that infants tend to sway and fall when the walls around them are suddenly moved, even though the platform they are standing on remains stationary. The visual information which is in conflict with vestibular and kinesthetic feedback gives rise to an inappropriate postural adjustment. Bower *et al.* (1970) found that visual inputs have better control over the prehensile system than do tactile-kinesthetic inputs in the absence of vision.

In contrast to these developmental studies, several recent adult studies support the idea that visual dominance may depend upon how the subject allocates his attention. Warren and Cleaves (1971) found that the occurrence of visual dominance in spatial localization depends upon the degree of conflict. With small amounts of conflict ($10°$), which the subject may not notice, visual dominance was obtained. However, with large amounts of conflict ($40°-60°$) they found a reversal of the dominance effect in some conditions. Similarly, Miller (1972) found that the occurrence of visual dominance in a size judgment depends upon the subject's knowledge of the discrepancy. Subjects who were misled into believing that they were examining the same object with vision and touch showed the traditional visual dominance result. Those who were told they were examining two different objects (as in fact they were) did not. These results suggest that when the subject is aware of the discrepancy he can focus his attention on the kinesthetic information and visual dominance may not be obtained.

Several studies of prism adaptation strengthen this suggestion. Hay and Pick (1966) found that extensive exposure to movement of the whole body (rather than just one arm or hand) leads to a recalibration of the visual system instead of the kinesthetic system. Other investigators (Canon, 1970; Kelso *et al.*, 1975) manipulated attention more directly. It was found that the modality which undergoes recalibration depends almost entirely upon the locus of the subject's attention during exposure. In the absence of attentional manipulation, attention seems to be focused on vision; thus kinesthesis is recalibrated (Harris, 1965).

I recently designed an experiment (Klein, 1974a) to determine whether the visual dominance observed in reaction time (Jordan, 1972; Klein and Posner, 1974, exp. III) results from an attentional bias, or from a wired-in relationship between vision, kinesthesis, and attention. I first showed that if the subject did bias his attention toward a modality, his RT to unexpected stimuli in another modality would be increased. Given this result, it is possible to detect and/or discourage a bias of attention. In the earlier studies subjects knew in advance when they would receive a bimodal input. Suppose, however, that the subject is in a mixed-block condition in which a trial may consist of a visual movement, a kinesthetic movement, or a bimodal movement. If dominance is wired in, it should be obtained on the bimodal trials from these mixed blocks. If the subject biases his attention this can be measured by comparing visual and kinesthetic RT in this condition with that in pure blocks in which the subject knows the modality of the stimulus. Lastly, if the mixed-block condition discourages the subject from biasing his attention, and dominance is due to a bias, then it should not be found in this condition. Subjects were run in both pure and mixed blocks so that an assessment of a bias could be made. The data are shown in Table I. The visual dominance effect in the pure blocks is smaller than in previous experiments (13 msec), but is nevertheless significant. More important, the effect completely reverses in the mixed blocks (bimodal is faster than kinesthetic). Thus visual dominance in reaction time is not wired in. It seems to result from a bias to attend vision when a bimodal input is expected.

What might be the origin of the bias toward vision? At least two explanations are possible. Many of our movements are based on visual feedback. During such movements visual information is processed and corrections are issued to the

Table I
Performance in Pure and Mixed Blocks[a,b,c]

Stimulus	Pure blocks		Mixed blocks	
	RT	Errors (%)	RT	Errors (%)
Visual	317	2.9	337	1.8
Kinesthetic	248	4.0	260	10.7
Bimodal	261	4.6	243	7.9

[a]From Klein (1974a).
[b]Reaction time is in milliseconds.
[c]The difference between visual and bimodal RT in the pure blocks seems inconsistent with visual dominance. Differences in error rates, however, suggest that the RT difference may be due to an alerting effect of the kinesthetic input in the bimodal condition.

muscles on the basis of this feedback. Kinesthetic information which is present need not be monitored at a conscious level during such visually guided movements (although there is no evidence that it is not). Perhaps a tendency to attend vision and ignore kinesthesis while watching the limbs becomes habitual and automatic. An alternative proposal has been made by Posner et al. (1975). The bias to attend vision may have its origins in the different alerting capabilities of the two modalities: Visual inputs seem to be inferior in activating attention. For example, if one does not attend vision, responses to visual inputs will suffer in latency and, if they are brief, may be missed altogether. We may develop a strategy of attending vision in order to counteract this deficiency. This view has an ironic twist: Visual dominance may result from a strategy developed to overcome the relative impotence of visual inputs for activating attention.

IV. Production of Movement

A. Introduction

When you first learn a new skill it seems to be performed properly only with a great deal of concentration and effort. With practice the skill is performed with a decreasing involvement of attention, until it seems to be performed automatically (effortlessly). Are these common introspections correct? If so, how does the change take place? What functions does attention perform in the production of movement? What will be the consequences if attention is not allocated when it is required? These questions are of practical and theoretical importance in human performance. Although we do not have any definite answers, I think the secondary task technique can provide objective measurements that will greatly improve our understanding of the role of attention in the production of movement.

At the turn of the century psychologists found that mental activity interfered with simple motor performance such as the repetitive squeezing of a rubber ball (Binet, 1890) or the exertion of maximal force (Welch, 1898). Interest then was primarily with the attention demands of different types of mental activity. These seminal results, however, show that even the simplest of motor acts may require attention. In recent years the secondary task technique has been used in a variety of ways to study directly the role of attention in motor skills. It has been used as a probe to measure the attention demands of skills under different conditions (Brown, 1962; Michon, 1966; Barhick et al., 1954) or to measure the demands of component processes within a particular task (Posner and Keele, 1969; Ells, 1973; Kerr, 1975). In contrast, the secondary task technique has also been used to occupy the subject's attention, to determine if a particular skill can be performed automatically, or to determine which aspects of the skill do not suffer from the withdrawal of attention (Posner, 1971; Pew, 1974).

B. Analysis of Speeded Responses: What Takes Attention?

Movements are often made in response to environmental stimulation. Psychologists have devised a wide range of tasks to study the processes that intervene between a stimulus and the response to a stimulus. The most frequently used paradigm is one in which the subject must make one of several simple responses contingent upon the identity of the stimulus presented. In this type of reaction time task, several operations have been assumed to intervene between the stimulus and the response. On the basis of studies of the psychological refractory period (PRP)[5] (Karlin and Kestenbaum, 1968) and converging evidence from other areas Keele (1973) has argued that response initiation requires attention while the complex and often time-consuming operations that precede it such as memory retrieval and response selection do not. This assertion has important implications for human performance because response initiation and response selection are frequent components of many skills. In this section I will point out some interesting exceptions to Keele's assertion. These exceptions suggest that we have to do more research and thinking before we will have a complete account of what takes attention in speeded responses to input signals.[6]

There are two types of study which demonstrate that response selection may require attention. In some studies of the PRP (Bertelson and Tisseyre, 1969; Ells, 1973; Smith, 1967) the subject makes a response to one value of the first stimulus, and refrains from responding to the other value. If response initiation requires attention but selecting a response does not, then there should be a delay in the response to the second stimulus only when there is a response to the first one. Although these studies found less interference when the first stimulus did

---

[5] In a typical PRP task the subject might be presented with a visual and an auditory signal separated by a variable interval (ISI). Each stimulus requires a response (e.g., a 2-choice discrimination). In most situations RT to the second stimulus is greater at short ISIs than at long ones. This delay at short ISIs is referred to as the PRP effect.

[6] Chapter 5 (Time and Attention in Retrieving Information from Memory) from Keele's book (1973) is highly recommended. Evidence from a variety of reaction time paradigms is covered and a general model of memory retrieval ("logogen" model) is presented to account for this corpus of data. This model clearly illustrates the concept of response conflict which I make reference to in this section. It should also be pointed out that while Keele does conclude that "memory retrieval does not take attention while response initiation does [p. 108]" his main point is that the activation of memory representations (including responses) following presentation of a stimulus is automatic while subsequent operations performed upon these representations may require attention. This view can accommodate the exceptions discussed below. One need only assume that on some occasions the memory retrieval stage does not produce a clearly defined response. On such occasions subsequent mental operations such as active search or comparison would demand attention. If correct, this theoretical extension suggests that we should try to specify the conditions which are necessary for the memory retrieval stage to produce a clearly defined response.

not require a response, the interference in this situation was still significant. This suggests that the decision not to respond requires attention. The difference between the two conditions shows that the initiation of the response requires additional attention. The conclusion that response selection may require attention seems unavoidable unless one makes the awkward assumption that the subject initiates a suppressive response when none is required.

Keele (1967) found more interference between two tasks where one involved incompatible stimulus-response (S-R) mappings than when it did not. Since Keele (1973) attributes the effects of S-R compatibility to memory retrieval stages, this result is contrary to his view. He suggests that practice may be a crucial factor. At low levels of practice (as in the 1967 study) compatibility may affect attention demands. Such an assumption points toward a more dynamic view of skill learning and attention. Some aspect of the memory retrieval stage may require attention when the S-R mapping is incompatible. I suggest that attention may be needed to resolve competition among simultaneous response tendencies. The degree of competition is high with incompatible mappings but decreases with practice. If and when it is eliminated there may be no demands upon attention.

If correct, this view suggests that response initiation itself may not require attention when the S-R mapping is very direct, or the S-R sequence is highly overlearned. Highly overlearned and compatible S-R mappings may be initiated so quickly (Evarts, 1973; Leonard, 1959; Seibel, 1963) that one might conclude that attention is not involved (Klein and Posner, 1974). However, as Keele points out, while time may index some aspects of difficulty, it does not necessarily reflect attentional requirements. Several studies have examined the attention demands of highly compatible or highly overlearned S-R mappings. Gottsdanker and Stelmach (1971) examined the PRP effect as a function of practice. Although the interference was significantly reduced, it was not completely eliminated even after 80 sessions. Since the two stimuli were visual it might be argued that the residual interference was structural rather than attentional. Greenwald and Schulman (1973) used extremely compatible S-R mappings (they use the term ideomotor compatibility) in a PRP situation. The first task was to move a lever in the direction of a visually displayed arrow, and the second task was to repeat a letter (either a or b) presented aurally. The PRP effect was eliminated in this condition. Supporting evidence that response initiation may be automatic when the S-R mapping is very direct comes from a study by Noble et al. (1967). They examined manual tracking performance during a variety of simultaneous tasks. When the subject was learning a list of digits by the serial anticipation method there was a significant decrement in tracking performance (compared to tracking with no other task). However, the decrement was no greater than when the subject was only required to freely produce digits (vocalize, with the restriction of no repetitions) suggesting that the demands are not associated with learning (see McLeod, 1973, for a critical discussion of this conclusion). Is the selection of the response (decision) or its initiation demanding? In another condition subjects were only required to repeat digits as they were presented over headphones (i.e., no selection was required). In this condition there was *no* decrement in tracking (see also McLeod, 1973, Figure 2). Thus selecting the digit to be articulated is attention demanding while the articulation itself is not. The process of selecting a response from a set of alternatives involves the reduction of competition between the responses. It seems intuitively appealing that when the input signal strongly activates only one response because of practice and/or compatibility, the attention demands of the selection process may be substantially reduced.

C. Attention Demands of Simple Movements

Since most movements last longer than the speeded responses discussed in the previous section, what we can learn about motor control from studies of such responses is rather limited. In this section I will discuss studies of the attention demands of relatively simple movements which are usually aimed at a target.

Posner and Keele (1969) were the first to attempt to map out the attentional requirements of simple movements. Their subjects rotated a handle (using a wrist rotation) to move a pointer to a target location. On two-thirds of the trials an auditory signal was presented (over headphones) at specific positions during the movement. The subject was to respond as quickly as possible to this signal with his other hand without interrupting the movement. In a control condition the subject responded to the auditory probe while no movement was made. The amount of attention required by the movement was determined for each probe position by subtracting probe RT in the control condition from that obtained during the movement.

In the first experiment the subject was required to move the pointer to a large or small target. The results of this experiment are shown in Figure 2a. It can be seen that the initiation of the movement requires considerable attention, and the demands at this position do not seem to be related to the required accuracy. The attention required during the course of the movement decreases after the movement is initiated and rises again near the termination of the movement. The attention demands are greater for the entire course of the movement when greater accuracy (small target) is required.

In a second experiment the demands of four different types of movements were compared. The movements were either visually guided, or blind. The visually guided movements were either to a clearly marked target (external) or to a remembered visual location (internal). For the blind movements the subject would move until he encountered a mechanical stop (external) or he had to

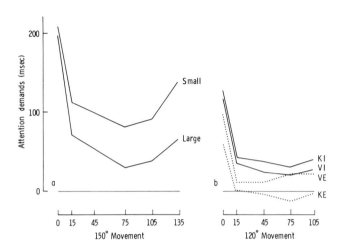

Figure 2 Attention demands during simple movements. Attention demands (probe RT during movement minus probe RT without movement) as a function of type of movement and position in the movement. (a) Movements to a large or small target. (b) Visually guided movements to a remembered location (VI) or a visible target (VE). Blind movements to a remembered location (KI) or a mechanical stop (KE). (Data are replotted from Posner and Keele, 1969.)

terminate the movement prior to the stop (internal). The attention demands were evaluated as in the previous experiment and are shown in Figure 2b. The demands are generally lower than in the previous study. This is probably due to differences in practice. The demands during the visual external condition are similar to that in the first experiment. They are high at the initiation of the movement and there is a slight upswing at the end. Data from the internal conditions (KI and VI) show that moving to a target stored in memory requires additional attention. The blind movements to a mechanical stop (KE) demand no attention once they are initiated. Thus, moving per se does not always require attention.

Ells (1973) varied the directional uncertainty and required accuracy of visually guided movements. Attention demands during the initiation and the movement agree with the notion (Fitts and Peterson, 1964) that movement selection and movement execution are independent processes. In most respects Ells' probe data agree with those of Posner and Keele. Two differences, however, should be mentioned. First, movements to a large target required almost no attention. These were completed so quickly (156 msec) that visual feedback could not have been used (see Keele and Posner, 1968). Ells' subjects apparently learned to execute a ballistic movement which gets the pointer to the large target without much attention. Second, Ells failed to find an increase in attention demands as the movement approached the target. One explanation for this discrepancy has to do with whether the subjects were allowed to make corrections when they overshot the target. Ells found weak support for this idea. A more plausible explanation is suggested by a close look at how the probe task was presented in the two studies. Ells presented a probe on every trial, while Posner and Keele presented probes only on two thirds of the trials. When a probe occurs on every trial the probability of a probe occurrence approaches 1.0 as the movement progresses. The subjects may develop an expectancy that would lead to reduced RT late in the movement, thus cancelling the increase. This explanation is supported by Salmoni (1972) who found an increase with the probe presented on five-eighths of the trials, but not when it was presented on every trial.

Often during a movement it is necessary to process information which will influence the future course of the movement. Kerr (1975) studied the attention demands associated with such processing. Her subjects guided a stylus through a semicircular track. In some conditions there was a choice of paths at the end of the track, in others there was no choice. When there was a choice, the subject was informed of the correct path at different stages during the movement. When the subject begins the movement without knowing the final destination, movement time and attention demands are increased. Kerr suggests that the high attention demands might be due to a focusing of attention on the expected informative signal. An interesting aspect of Kerr's data is that even when there is no choice concerning the path, the movement requires considerable attention. On the surface this movement resembles a blind movement to a stop so one might expect it to be performed automatically. Kerr discusses several possible explanations for the attentional demands of this semicircular movement. One is that the semicircular movement requires a change in prime movers midway through the movement, while the movements in the previous studies do not. Another explanation is based on how the different movements were constrained. In the previous experiments (Posner and Keele, 1969; Ells, 1973) the movements were constrained by the apparatus. That is, the subject moved a lever or handle with only one degree of freedom. These movements could be made by the application of sufficient force for the stop to be reached. In Kerr's situation the subject has to keep the point of a stylus in a groove. The fact that the subject occasionally made errors by leaving the track shows that this movement could not be accomplished simply by the application of force. In order to stay in the track the subject probably has to monitor tactile-kinesthetic feedback and make corrections based on this feedback. This comparison suggests that truly automated movements may occur only in very limited situations.

Posner (1971) used a related method to determine whether different types of repetitive movements could be performed automatically. Highly practiced subjects were instructed to move rhythmically between stops, between visual targets, or between remembered targets without vision. Two continuous secondary tasks were used to occupy the subject's attention. One task involved maintaining the position of a telegraph key. For the other task the subject was merely asked to think about something else. The rhythmic movements were performed alone and with each secondary task. Movement time, pause time and movement distance were examined, with special emphasis placed upon variability of these parameters. The "key" task increased variability for all three types of movements. The "think" task had a similar, but nonsignificant effect. Since a single movement to a stop can be performed automatically we might ask why the repetitive movement between stops was affected by the simultaneous tasks. A likely explanation follows from the fact that even for blind movements to a stop movement initiation requires attention (see Figure 2). This view is supported by the finding that the simultaneous tasks caused a greater increase in pause time variability than in movement time variability. Another interesting finding was that movement distance variability in the blind task without stops increased only slightly when attention was withdrawn. This finding converges with some evidence suggesting that the retention of kinesthetic distance cues is not much affected by attentional manipulations (Posner, 1967; Laabs, 1973).

The studies described above begin to provide a picture of the time course of the attention demands during movement. The question, what processes require attention? still remains. Keele (1968) has proposed that a visually guided movement is composed of an initial movement toward the target, and a series of corrections based upon visual feedback. This view was developed to explain the relationship between movement size, target size, and movement time described by Fitts' Law (Fitts, 1954). If it is assumed (see Keele, 1973, Chapter 6) that the initiation of each correction requires attention (as the initiation of the original movement does) then the pattern of attention demands discussed above fits nicely with Keele's feedback interpretation. For example, the upswing near the target occurs because more corrections are made as the subject approaches the target. When the size of the target decreases attention demands increase because the number of corrections increases. A movement to a mechanical stop should not require any attention after its initiation, because no corrections are necessary.

An alternative to this view is that the attention demands are associated with the monitoring of feedback and not the initiation of corrections. None of the studies discussed so far have separated these alternatives. There are some suggestions that merely monitoring sensory information without responding to it does not require attention. Salmoni (1974) examined the variability of the speed of handle-cranking while subjects monitored vision, kinesthesis or both modalities. Variability was not greater in the dual modality monitoring condition. Similarly, Shiffrin and Grantham (1974) have shown that sensitivity (d') is equal whether the subject is attending one or three modalities. These results are only suggestive, however, because the information monitored is unlike that used in the control of movement.

D. Attention Demands during Pursuit Tracking:
A Model Situation

Understanding the attention demands associated with visually guided motor behavior is of great practical and theoretical significance. Many motor skills involve the use of visual feedback and the data discussed above suggest that some components of visually guided movement require attention. One task that has been widely used as a prototype for visual-motor skills is pursuit tracking. In this task the subject follows the movement of a target on a screen with a cursor which he controls by moving a lever. His goal is to minimize the distance (error) between the target and the cursor. The movement of the target may be one- or two-dimensional, simple or complex; its velocity may be constant or vary continuously; the predictability of its course can be manipulated.

While tracking the subject intermittently makes small corrections as he drifts off target (Vince, 1948). When the target changes direction a large correction is required. I performed several experiments to explore the following questions: (1) What are the attention demands of merely tracking a target? (2) Will the demands following target reversals be reduced if the subject knows when and where the reversal will occur? In these experiments the target motion was in a horizontal direction and its velocity was constant. The path of the target was computer controlled and the subject's performance was monitored and selectively recorded on magnetic tape for later analysis.

In one experiment[7] (Klein and Posner, 1974, exp. IV) a continuous tracking task was used. The subject tracked a moving target for 5-min intervals (blocks) during which occasional auditory tones were presented. The subject responded to these tones with his other hand. The target could only reverse directions at five fixed locations (which were not marked on the screen). Whether or not a reversal occurred when the target passed one of these locations was determined randomly. Naturally, reversals had to occur at the two exterior locations (end points). Thus reversals at the three interior locations were always unpredictable, while those at the end points could be anticipated. The auditory probes were presented unpredictably at delays of 50, 150, and 250 msec following some of the expected and unexpected reversals. Probes were also presented at the same delays after the target passed an interior location without reversing. In control blocks the subject responded to the probes while simply watching the target. The demands of tracking were determined by subtracting probe RTs obtained during watching from those during tracking. This procedure controls for the subject's ability to use the target motion to predict the occurrence of a probe.

Tracking performance is shown in Figure 3. In the absence of a reversal

---

[7] This experiment was discussed briefly by Klein and Posner (1974). In this chapter I present the results in greater detail.

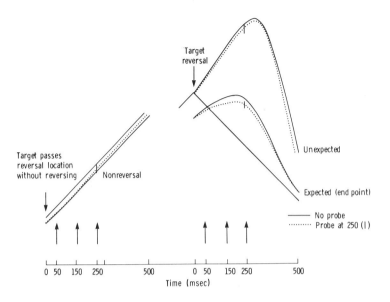

Figure 3 Tracking performance from a continuous pursuit task. The solid straight lines show target position (ordinate) as a function of time (abscissa). The solid and dotted curves show cursor position averaged across 6 subjects. Upward pointing arrows mark the times at which probes were presented. See text for explanation and Table II for attention demands.

subjects generally lag the target. When a reversal unexpectedly occurs the error increases as the subject continues to move in an inappropriate direction. The subject begins to make a correction in about 200–300 msec which is usually completed within 600 msec of the target reversal. When the subject expects the target to reverse his performance is much better: The maximum error is smaller and the return to target faster. It can be seen that a decrease in velocity begins before the target reversal. The occurrence of a probe had little effect on tracking performance (dotted line).

Attention demands are shown in Table II. An analysis of variance reveals a significant effect of tracking condition but no effect of delay and no delay condition interaction. All conditions require attention (i.e., the scores are significantly greater than zero) and all the conditions differ at the 0.05 level (expected and unexpected differ at the 0.01 level). Is the amount of attention required in the absence of a reversal related to the size of the correction which must be made at the time of the probe? The correlation between probe RT and tracking error at the time of the probe was calculated to answer this question. Averaged over subjects and delays, this correlation is extremely small (0.10), indicating that the attention demands of nonreversal tracking are not necessarily related to correction size. The attention demands following reversals did not seem to be

Table II
Attention Demands (RT-Tracking Minus
RT-Watching, msec) in a Continuous Tracking Task

Condition	Probe position (msec)			
	+50	+150	+250	Mean
Unexpected reversal	39	21	29	29
Expected reversal	49	48	58	52
Nonreversal	41	38	43	41

affected by delay. This might be due to the narrow range of probe delays used. Contrary to expectation, the demands following an unexpected reversal were less than those following an expected reversal. Thus the improved tracking performance in the expected condition is accomplished at the expense of the processing of other signals. My tentative interpretation of this surprising finding is that knowing in advance when and where the target will reverse allows the subject to minimize his error only if he pays close attention to the tracking task. When an unexpected reversal occurs the subject can do little besides initiate a gross correction which requires little attention.

One problem with this experiment is that the expected reversals were always at end points. The difference in attention demands might be due to this feature instead of predictability. In two further experiments (Klein, 1974b) a discrete trials procedure was used to eliminate this confounding. The target moved from the left side of the screen to a reversal location, reversed direction, and returned to the starting position. On one-half of the trials the subject could not anticipate the reversal. On the remaining trials the subject was informed in advance of the trial which reversal location would be used. In one experiment this was accomplished by marking the location on the screen with pointers, while in the other the subject was shown a number indicating the location. As we shall see this difference has profound consequences. A 2-choice auditory probe was presented occasionally at various positions.

The results of the first experiment are shown in Figure 4 and Table III. The previous finding was not replicated: probe RT at the +50 and +350 msec delays was actually faster for the expected reversals (errors are in the same direction). Tracking performance in the expected condition is remarkably accurate. It may be that the clearly marked location in combination with the discrete nature of this task enabled the subjects to execute a preprogrammed reversal which is timed to coincide with the target reversal. The execution of this program may require little or no attention once it is initiated. In light of this speculation it is interesting to note that 700 msec prior to the reversal probe RT in the expected

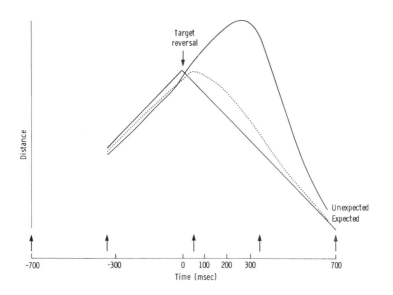

Figure 4 Tracking performance from a discrete task. Solid straight line shows target position as a function of time. The solid and dotted curves show cursor position averaged across 5 subjects. Upward pointing arrows mark the times at which probes occurred. In this experiment expected reversals were clearly marked on the scope. See text for explanation and Table III for probe data.

condition is greater than in the unexpected condition. This might reflect the attention demands of initiating the preprogrammed reversal.

In the second experiment an attempt was made to more closely simulate the expected reversal tracking performance of the continuous task. On the expected trials the location was not marked on the scope, but instead the subject was shown a digit (1–4) telling him at which of the four locations the target would reverse. The results are shown in Figure 5 and Table IV. A comparison with

Table III
Probe RT (msec) in a Discrete Tracking Task

Condition	Probe position (msec)				
	−700	−350	+50	+350	+700
Unexpected reversal	449	455	556	506	461
Expected reversal	493	461	496	460	469

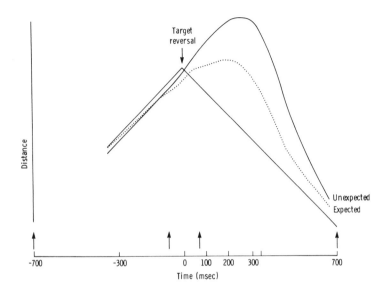

Figure 5 Tracking performance from a discrete task. Solid straight line shows target position as a function of time. The solid and dotted curves show cursor position averaged across 5 subjects. Upward pointing arrows mark the times at which probes occurred. In this experiment expected reversals were not clearly marked on the scope. See text for explanation and Table IV for attention demands.

Figure 3 shows that the tracking performance in the expected condition was similar to that of the continuous task. Attention demands for the two conditions differ only at 70 msec prior to the reversal.[8] As in the continuous task the expected reversal requires more attention than the unexpected reversal. The

Table IV
Attention Demands (RT-Tracking Minus RT-Watching,
msec) in a Discrete Tracking Task

	Probe position (msec)			
Condition	−700	−70	+70	+700
Unexpected reversal	135	102	193	101
Expected reversal	150	197	212	97

[8] That no difference is found at +70 is a problem. It may be explained by assuming that the discrete task allows a finer discrimination of the time-course of the attention demands or that the time-course is somewhat different in the discrete task.

original difference cannot be attributed to end points being somehow different from interior reversals, because in this experiment both expected and unexpected reversals occurred at the same locations.

These studies show that tracking itself requires attention. Although planning or preparing a correction (reversal) usually requires additional attention, in some situations the subject may execute a preprogrammed movement sequence which requires little attention. These studies of attention demands during movement demonstrate the importance of strategies and the findings fit nicely with the view of attention outlined in Section II,B. Attention does not seem to be tightly tied to a specific aspect of visually guided motor control: It seems to be allocated flexibly depending upon the nature of the task.

E. Observations on the Attention Demands of Skills

Our own introspections suggest that repetitive tasks may be performed automatically. Barhick (Barhick *et al.*, 1954; Barhick and Shelley, 1958) has explored the effects of practice and redundancy upon the attention demands of a visual serial reaction task. In one study (Barhick *et al.*, 1954) subjects responded to a fixed or random sequence of stimuli. A simultaneous secondary task (mental arithmetic) was performed either early or late in practice. The results suggest that the attention demands of a repetitive serial reaction task decrease only after the subject learns about the predictability of the sequence. It could not be determined if the repetitive task was performed automatically because mental arithmetic was not tested alone.

In a second study Barhick and Shelley (1958) used a difficult secondary task (auditory serial reactions with the other hand). Surprisingly, performance on the secondary auditory task was unaffected by the redundancy or level of practice of the primary task. Performance on the primary task alone was at asymptote by the second session, and the different levels of redundancy could not be distinguished because of the ceiling effect. However, when the two tasks were performed simultaneously primary task performance deteriorated. The amount of deterioration was inversely related to the amount of practice and redundancy. Even after twenty five sessions the auditory task interfered with the primary task. A structural explanation for this interference is contradicted by the fact that at all levels of practice the degree of interference is a function of redundancy. It seems that some component of the serial reaction task cannot be automated. Barhick and Shelley suggest that the reduced interference at high levels of practice and redundancy is due to a transfer from visual to kinesthetic control of the response sequence. The data in Figure 2b (From Posner and Keele, 1969), however, show that kinesthetic control is not necessarily less demanding than visual control (KI versus VI). The reduced attentional requirements could be due to the learning of a motor program (Keele, 1968) or to the reduction of response uncertainty.

An interesting study by Pew (1974) demonstrates that repetition and practice are not always accompanied by a decreased involvement of attention. He found that performance in compensatory tracking improved faster (over 16 sessions) for a repeating segment than for nonrepeating segments even when subjects were unaware of the repetition. A secondary task (memory load) was used to assess attention. It was found that the subjects were allocating more attention to the repeating segment, and performance on the repeating segment was more adversely affected by distraction than performance on the nonrepeated segments. With Pew's task, improved performance on a repeating pattern is accomplished only with the allocation of additional attention. This finding may be related to the results of my studies of pursuit tracking (Section IV,D). When the subject in the pursuit task knows what to expect he performs better and usually allocates more attention to tracking. The trend is similar in Pew's experiment, even though several of his subjects were not aware of the repetition.

The secondary task technique has not been restricted to laboratory experiments on "artificial" skills. Brown (1962), for example, used an auditory task to assess the demands of automobile driving. As one might expect, it was found that driving in a residential area requires less attention than driving in a busy shopping area. Since the auditory task was not timed to occur during particular operations it could not be determined which aspects of driving (increased perceptual load; increased number of responses, e.g., braking, acceleration, gear changes; or increased accuracy required in maneuvering) impose greater demands in the shopping area. By carefully timing the secondary task to overlap specific primary task components a fine-grained description of the attention demands of a motor skill can be achieved.

Even when the placement of the probe task is not controlled, the secondary task technique can provide very useful data. For instance, Klonoff (1974) recently examined the effects of marijuana on driving performance. Although most subjects' performance deteriorated under the influence of marijuana, a few subjects actually showed an improvement. Klonoff concluded that "whether or not a significant decline occurs in driving ability is dependent upon the subject's ability to compensate." Within the framework of this chapter Klonoff's *post hoc* conclusion suggests that some subjects allocate more attention to driving when they know they are "stoned." Secondary task measures of attention could have provided direct evidence to support or contradict this interpretation. If, as I have suggested, attention can be allocated by the subject in varying degrees, then it is essential that attempts to measure the effects of stressors, drugs, and other variables upon performance be bolstered by probe measures of attention, so that the subject's strategic control over attention (which can influence performance markedly) may be monitored by the experimenter.

V. Conclusion

In this chapter I have discussed the role of attention in movement. In psychology a distinction is often made between action (movement) and perception. I think this distinction may obscure some common explanatory principles (see also Turvey, 1973). The study of attention reveals that there are, in fact, similarities between perception and action. For example, many perceptions and actions can be achieved automatically, while the achievement of others requires attention. Thus, the answer to the question "How do pathways in the nervous system become automated?" may apply equally to pathways leading to action and perception.

The value of a concept is often measured in terms of the range of phenomena to which it can be profitably applied. I think that the concepts we use to describe the acquisition and limitations of skilled performance in adults should also be useful in understanding performance at other developmental levels. The concept of attention adopted in this chapter may, in fact, be very useful for characterizing some features of infant behavior. Visual pursuit and sucking are motor responses which are in the infant's repertoire at birth, and which are often referred to as "reflexes." Wolff (1965) has observed that infants under 3 weeks of age cannot perform both activities (visual pursuit and sucking) at the same time. When an infant who is sucking on a nipple is shown a moving object, visual pursuit does not occur, unless the infant stops sucking. The same limitation is found when the infant is presented with a nipple while engaged in visual pursuit. After 3 weeks of age, however, the infant is able to perform both activities simultaneously. It is exciting to consider that the processes underlying this developmental change may be the same as those leading to the reduction of attention demands in adult performance.

References

Barhick, H.P., and Shelley, C. (1958). *J. Exp. Psychol.* **56**, 288–293.
Barhick, H.P., Noble, M., and Fitts, P.M. (1954). *J. Exp. Psychol.* **48**, 298–302.
Bertelson, P., and Tisseyre, F. (1969). *J. Exp. Psychol.* **79**, 122–128.
Binet, A. (1890). *Rev. Phil. Fr. Estranger* 24, 138–155.
Bower, T.G.R., Broughton, M., and Moore, M.K. (1970). *Percept. & Psychophys.* **8**, 51–53.
Brindley, K., and Merton, P.A. (1960). *J. Physiol. (London)* 153, 127–310.
Broadbent, D.E. (1958). "Perception and Communication." Pergamon, Oxford.
Brown, I.D. (1962). *Ergonomics* 5, 247–250.
Browne, K., Lee, J., and Ring, P.A. (1954). *J. Physiol. (London)* 15, 205–212.
Canon, L.K. (1970). *J. Exp. Psychol.* **84**, 141–147.
Corteen, R.S., and Wood, B. (1972). *J. Exp. Psychol.* **94**, 308–313.
Deutsch, J.A., and Deutsch, D. (1963). *Psychol. Rev.* **70**, 80–90.
Ells, J.G. (1973). *J. Exp. Psychol.* **99**, 10–21.

Evarts, E.V. (1971). *Neurosci. Res. Program, Bull.* **9**, 86–132.

Evarts, E.V. (1973). *Science* **179**, 501–503.

Evarts, E.V., and Tanji, J. (1974). *Brain Res.* **71**, 479–494.

Festinger, L., Ono, H., Burnham, C.A., and Bambar, D. (1967). *J. Exp. Psychol.* **74**, Monogr. No. 2, Part 2.

Fetz, E.E., and Finocchio, D.V. (1971). *Science* **174**, 431–435.

Fitts, P.M. (1954). *J. Exp. Psychol.* **47**, 481–391.

Fitts, P.M., and Peterson, J.R. (1964). *J. Exp. Psychol.* **65**, 423–432.

Gelfan, S., and Carter, S. (1967). *Exp. Neurol.* **18**, 469–473.

Gibson, J.J. (1943). *J. Exp. Psychol.* **16**, 1–31.

Goldscheider, S. (1889). *Arch. Anat. Physiol.* **Lpz. 13**, 369–502.

Goodwin, G., McCloskey, I., and Matthews, P. (1972). *Science* **175**, 1382–1384.

Gottsdanker, R., and Stelmach, G.E. (1971). *J. Mot. Behav.* **3**, 301–312.

Granit, R., and Burke, R. (1973). *Brain Res.* **53**, 1–28.

Greenwald, A.G., and Schulman, H.G. (1973). *J. Exp. Psychol.* **101**, 70–76.

Harris, C.S. (1965). *Psychol. Rev.* **72**, 419–444.

Hay, J.C., and Pick, H.L. (1966). *J. Exp. Psychol.* **71**, 150–158.

Hay, J.C., Pick, H.L., and Ikeda, K. (1965). *Psychonom. Sci.* **2**, 215–216.

Hernandes-Peon, R., Scherrer, H., and Jouvet, M. (1956). *Science* **123**, 331–332.

Howard, I.P., and Templeton, W.B. (1966). "Human Spatial Orientation." Wiley, New York.

James, W. (1890). "The Principles of Psychology." Holt, New York.

Jordan, T.C. (1972). *Quart. J. Exp. Psychol.* **24**, 536–543.

Kahneman, D. (1973). "Attention and Effort." Prentice-Hall, Englewood Cliffs, New Jersey.

Karlin, L., and Kestenbaum, R. (1968). *Quart. J. Exp. Psychol.* **20**, 447–451.

Keele, S.W. (1967). *J. Exp. Psychol.* **75**, 529–539.

Keele, S.W. (1968). *Psychol. Bull.* **70**, 387–403.

Keele, S.W. (1973). "Attention and Human Performance." Goodyear, Pacific Palisades, California.

Keele, S.W., and Posner, M.I. (1968). *J. Exp. Psychol.* **77**, 353–363.

Kelso, J.A.S., Cook, E., Olson, M.E., and Epstein, W. (1975). *Hum. Percept. & Perf.* **1**, 237–245.

Kerr, B. (1973). *Memory & Cognition* **1**, 401–412.

Kerr, B. (1975). *J. Mot. Behav.* **7**, 15–28.

Kinney, J.A.S., and Luria, S.M. (1970). *Percept. & Psychophys.* **8**, 189–192.

Klein, R.M. (1974a). Ph.D. Dissertation, University of Oregon, Eugene.

Klein, R.M. (1974b). *Pap., West. Psychol. Ass., 1974.*

Klein, R.M., and Posner, M.I. (1974). *Brain Res.* **71**, 401–411.

Klonoff, H. (1974). *Science* **186**, 317–324.

Laabs, G.J. (1973). *J. Exp. Psychol.* **100**, 168–177.

Laberge, D.H. (1975). *In* "Attention and Performance V" (P.M.A. Rabbitt and S. Dornic, eds.), Academic Press, New York.

Lashley, K. (1917). *Amer. J. Physiol.* **43**, 169–194.

Lee, D.N., and Aronson, E. (1974). *Percept. & Psychophys.* **15**, 529–532.

Leonard, J.A. (1959). *Quart. J. Exp. Psychol.* **11**, 76–83.

Lewis, J. (1970). *J. Exp. Psychol.* **85**, 225–226.

MacKay, D. (1966). *In* "Brain and Conscious Experience" (J.C. Eccles, ed.), pp. 422–445. Springer-Verlag, Berlin and New York.

MacKay, D.G. (1973). *Quart. J. Exp. Psychol.* **25**, 22–40.

McLeod, P.D. (1973). *J. Exp. Psychol.* **99**, 330–333.

Matthews, P.B.C. (1972). "Mammalian Muscle Receptors and Their Central Actions." Arnold, London.

Merton, P.A. (1964). *Symp. Soc. Exp. Biol.* **182**, 387–400.

Merton, P.A. (1972). *Sci. Amer.* **226**, 30–37.

Michon, J.A. (1966). *Ergonomics* **9**, 401–412.

Miller, E.A. (1972). *J. Exp. Psychol.* **96**, 114–123.

Milner, P. (1970). "Physiological Psychology." Holt, New York.

Moray, N. (1967). *Acta Psychol.* **27**, 84–92.

Moruzzi, G., and Magoun, H.W. (1949). *Electroencephalogr. Clin. Neurophysiol.* **1**, 445–473.

Nickerson, R. (1973). *Psychol. Rev.* **80**, 489–509.

Noble, M., Trumbo, D., and Fowler, F. (1967). *J. Exp. Psychol.* **73**, 146–149.

Norman, D.A. (1968). *Psychol. Rev.* **75**, 522–536.

Pew, R.W. (1974). *Brain Res.* **71**, 393–400.

Phillips, C.G. (1973). *Proc. Roy. Soc. Med.* **66**, 41–56.

Pick, H.L., Pick, A.D., and Klein, R.E. (1967). *Advan. Child Develop. Behav.* **3**, 190–223.

Pick, H.L., Warren, D.H., and Hay, J.C. (1969). *Percept. & Psychophys.* **6**, 203–205.

Posner, M.I. (1967). *J. Exp. Psychol.* **75**, 103–107.

Posner, M.I. (1971). *J. Mot. Behav.* **1**, 245–258.

Posner, M.I., and Boies, S.W. (1971). *Psychol. Rev.* **78**, 391–408.

Posner, M.I., and Keele, S.W. (1969). *Proc. Congr. Appl. Psychol., 17th, 1968* pp. 412–422.

Posner, M.I., and Klein, R.M. (1973). *In* "Attention and Performance IV" (S. Kornblum, ed.), pp. 21–36. Academic Press, New York.

Posner, M.I., and Snyder, C.R.R. (1975a). *In* "Attention and Performance V" (P.M.A. Rabitt and S. Dornic, eds.), pp. 669–681. Academic Press, New York.

Posner, M.I., and Synder, C.R.R. (1975b). *In* "Information Processing and Cognition: The Loyola Symposium" (R. Solso, ed.). Erlbaum, New York.

Posner, M.I., Nissen, M.J., and Klein, R.M. (1976). *Psychol. Rev.* (in press).

Provins, K.A. (1958). *J. Physiol. (London)* **143**, 55–67.

Rock, I., and Victor, J. (1964). *Science* **143**, 594–596.

Rock, I., Mack, A., Adams, L., and Hill, L. (1965). *Psychonom. Sci.* **3**, 435–436.

Salmoni, A.W. (1972). *Proc. Can. Symp. Psycho-Mot. Learn. Sports Psychol., 4th, 1972.*

Salmoni, A.W. (1974). Ph.D. Dissertation, University of Michigan, Ann Arbor.

Seibel, R. (1963). *J. Exp. Psychol.* **66**, 215–226.

Shallice, T. (1972). *Psychol. Rev.* **79**, 383–393.

Shiffrin, R.M., and Grantham D.W. (1974). *Percept. & Psychophys.* **15**, 460–474.

Skavensky, A. (1972). *Vision Res.* **12**, 221–229.

Smith, M.C. (1967). *Quart. J. Exp. Psychol.* **19**, 350–352.

Tastevin, J. (1937). *Encephale* **1**, 57–84 and 140–158.

Titchner, E.B. (1908). "Lectures on the Elementary Psychology of Feeling and Attention." Macmillan, New York.

Turvey, M.T. (1973). *In* "Psychology of Motor Behavior and Sport," pp. 71–76. Univ. of Illinois Press, Urbana.

Vince, M.A. (1948). *Quart. J. Exp. Psychol.* **1**, 85–103.

Walker, J.T. (1972). *Percept. & Psychophys.* **11**, 247–251.

Warren, D.H., and Cleaves, W.T. (1971). *J. Exp. Psychol.* **90**, 206–214.

Warren, D.H., and Pick, H.L. (1970). *Percept. & Psychophys.* **8**, 430–433.

Welch, J.C. (1898). *Amer. J. Physiol.* **1**, 253–306.

Wolff, P.H. (1965). *Ann. N.Y. Acad. Sci.* **118**, 815–830.

Woodworth, R.S. (1899). *Psychol. Rev. Monogr., Suppl.* **3**, No. 13.

Cognitive Information Processes in Motor Short-Term Memory and Movement Production

Ronald G. Marteniuk

I. Introduction

As Broadbent (1971) has outlined, a shift in emphasis in the experimental study of human behavior has occurred over the past ten to fifteen years. Initially there was a primary concentration upon the relation between an isolated stimulus event and its corresponding motor event; although there were several variations of this theme (e.g., *Gestalt* psychology), a stimulus-response bond was thought to underlie all behavior. A second general theme arose in the 1950s when man was treated as a communciation channel, in a similar manner to a telephone, and where the correlation between stimulus and response was the main independent variable. In essence, man's capacity to process information was studied and, in general, it was found that he was a limited information processor.

While both these approaches have produced a voluminous amount of literature and have undoubtedly contributed much to understanding human behavior, they are ultimately limited in their ability to uncover the underlying causes of behavior. For instance, at the base of both these approaches is the view of behavior as being controlled by processes resembling reflex arcs. In addition,

175

comparing men to a limited communication channel seems highly inapprorpriate when studying the highly skilled and flexible behavior of a performer at advanced stages of learning whether it be verbal or motor in nature.

The third notion, while not new since its roots are in early psychology, is becoming fashionable and centers around the concept that an individual actively interacts with and operates upon stimuli. This cognitive approach to the study of behavior, which also can be termed an information-processing approach, is involved in following information through the processing system and determining, as exactly as possible, the various transformations the sensory input undergoes as it is processed by the central nervous system. Questions such as how an individual transforms or codes a stimulus, how he abstracts some features from it and neglects others, how he uses the coded information to modify some internal representation of the external world, how he manipulates this internal representation to symbolize events in space and time, and how he uses it to organize, initiate, and control movement are all of interest to a cognitive information-processing approach to the study of motor behavior.

While all these processes are of interest, I wish to concentrate exclusively upon the issue of coding and retention of movement information. The storage of information in memory is the first subprocess that forms the basis for all subsequent information-processing activities and thus its study would seem to be a prerequisite to understanding all skilled behavior. In essence, then, I wish to examine how an individual operates on movement information (i.e., cognitively manipulates it) so that it can be retained for short intervals, and how he eventually transforms this information into a more permanent form.

II. Coding Processes
in Motor Short-Term Memory

Over the past several years there have been various studies concerned with attempting to uncover those codes thought to underlie the retention of movement information. Perhaps the most systematic study done in this area was one by Laabs (1973) where he investigated the precision and retention characteristics of location, distance, and timing information. His blindfolded subjects were required to reproduce the end location or the distance of a standard movement where the starting location of the reproduction movement was made unreliable by randomly altering it. For example, if a subject was asked to reproduce the end location of the standard movement, distance cues were unreliable and hence only location cues could be used. Similarly, if the distance of the standard movement had to be reproduced, the end location of the standard movement became unreliable and the subject could only rely on distance cues. In the analysis of his results, Laabs also included, in a separate group, those subjects who admitted to using counting as an aid in movement reproduction. It was thought that counting might lead to coding a blind movement in terms of its rate and execution time. Analysis of the data revealed that there was a differential retention effect for the three types of cues. The location and counters groups both demonstrated an ability to retain accuracy over a 12-sec unfilled interval while the distance group became significantly worse. It would appear from this, then, that subjects are unable to centrally code and retain distance information, whereas there appears to be some mechanism which allows this process to occur for location and timing information.

These findings, however, were partially replicated and partially refuted in a study by Marteniuk (1973). Using a design similar to that of Laabs (1973) it was found that both location and distance cues were retained over an unfilled retention interval of 10 sec. This study differs from that of Laabs not only in that distance cues were retained over an unfilled retention interval but also in that immediate reproduction of distance information seemed to supply less precise information as seen by reproduction being inferior when compared to the location group. Thus it appears from this study that even though location and distance information were capable of being centrally represented the forms which they took were different.

Another source of movement information, not generally included in the study of retention of movement information, arises from the motor commands or efference as they leave the higher centers. Perhaps the strongest support for the notion that efferent information can be stored and used in the reproduction of movement comes from Lashley's work (1917) on a human patient whose afferent nerves in the lower leg were destroyed. This individual could not detect passive movement but was able to reproduce leg movements that he had actively executed just as well as normal individuals.

One other way of studying the contrast between properties of efferent and afferent information is to compare the retention of movements that are actively and passively presented to subjects. Two such studies (Marteniuk, 1973; Jones, 1974) show that voluntary movement not only results in better immediate reproduction but that it is also retained better than passively induced movement. These results have been interpreted as meaning that efferent information about where a limb will go is much more reliable and codable than information about where the limb has gone. However, in both these studies there is a confounding effect in that efferent information per se is not the only difference between the active and passive conditions. The active subjects, since they had to not only initiate but also terminate their standard movements, presumably had to know a good deal more about the task than the passive subjects. This task related information may have led to a better "idea" of the task which could have resulted either in subjects visualizing or imaging the required movements or in subjects formulating "plans of action" that would facilitate retention of the executed movement. Regardless, if one adheres to the definition of efference as movement information arising from the motor commands as they leave the higher centers, imaging and planning are not part of this type of information. Thus, one might speculate that it is this higher order planning process that differentiates the voluntary and passive conditions in the above two studies.

One type of information that might give a higher order structure to movement information is what Posner (1969) refers to as an image. In reviewing the work of Adams and Dijkstra (1966) and Bilodeau *et al.* (1962) Posner makes a strong case for the view that the basic code by which movement-related information is stored in short-term memory might be that of an image. An image in this case would be a nonverbal, relatively direct representation of the stimulus which could possibly be in the form of a spatial map containing detailed information about the characteristics of movement. One study that offers support for an image serving as the basis for retention of simple movements is by Posner (1967). He studied the retention of movements made under two different feedback conditions: in the kinesthetic feedback condition the blindfolded subject moved his arm a standard distance and reproduced it while blindfolded, and a kinesthetic plus visual feedback condition involved the same procedures as the kinesthetic condition except the subjects could watch their hand while moving during the criterion movement. Under each of these two conditions the subjects were required either to reproduce the end location or the distance of the standard movement where in this latter condition the starting location of the reproduction movement was made unreliable by randomly altering it. In addition three retention conditions were studied: immediate reproduction; a 20-sec retention interval where the subjects just rested after presentation; and a 20-sec retention interval during which the subjects were required to classify digit pairs into high or low and odd or even.

With the immediate reproduction condition serving as a reference point, the results indicated that regardless of the feedback condition or whether subjects were recalling location or distance cues, significant forgetting occurred in the 20-sec retention interval where subjects had to classify digits. However, during the unfilled retention interval all groups demonstrated forgetting except for the visual-kinesthetic group that had to reproduce the end location of the criterion or standard movement. Posner (1967) felt these latter results were support for the notion that an image was used as the basis for retaining the movement information not only because of the very accurate movement reproductions but also by the fact that the subjects reported using imagery as a guide in retaining and reproducing the standard movement.

If an image is used as the code for movement information this might explain the superiority of location information (Laabs, 1973; Marteniuk, 1973) over distance information in that spatial location is more easily coded as an image representing a spatial map. In addition, it might also account for why voluntary movement, which it was argued might initially involve a subject generating an image, is superior to passive movement. One implication of this viewpoint is that proprioceptive information by itself cannot be coded and as a result would demonstrate spontaneous loss of information. In essence this would mean that in the absence of vision, or perhaps audition, which could act as recoding system, proprioceptive information is not capable of existing in memory. This in turn would imply that the store for proprioceptive information would be analogous to the short-term sensory storage found for vision and audition (Keele, 1973) where information is available for short periods of time but since it is uncoded, spontaneously decays. The only difference would be that the proprioceptive short-term sensory storage system would have a longer decay time, perhaps as long as 20 sec.

Support for this viewpoint comes from Posner's results (1967) where it was shown that the kinesthetic feedback group became worse at movement reproduction over both the filled and unfilled retention interval. Another study, which actually took as its starting point the results from Posner's study, examined the relationship between vision and kinesthesis in more detail (Connolly and Jones, 1970). These authors postulated that at the base of improvements in perceptual-motor skills is the ability for individuals to make accurate judgments about the equivalence or nonequivalence of sensory input to two or more sensory modalities. Specifically, they felt that an important aspect of the retention of movement information was the development of an integrated visual-kinesthetic store that not only served as the basis for making equivalence judgments between these two sensory systems but also could be used to transform information from one of the senses into a form usable by the other system.

In studying the characteristics of this integrated store as well as its ability to recode or transform information from one form to another, Connolly and Jones examined the ability of subjects to make intra- and intermodal comparisons of visually or kinesthetically presented line lengths. For visual intramodal comparisons the subject told the experimenter when an ever-increasing line length matched the previous visually presented line length, and for kinesthetic intramodal comparisons the blindfolded subject actively estimated the end location of the standard. For intermodal comparisons if the standard was presented visually, the subject reproduced the visual line length by moving his arm, without the aid of vision, and if the standard was kinesthetic he reproduced a visual line length in the same manner as in the visual intramodal comparison.

The results indicated that the intramodal conditions were more accurate than the intermodal conditions. Presumably this was so because comparisons within a sense do not require the transfer of information between senses which would be a more difficult task. In terms of the intermodal comparisons an asymmetry between the two conditions resulted. The visual-to-kinesthetic condition produced substantially more error than the kinesthetic-to-visual condition. To account for this latter finding the authors postulated that in an intermodal matching task the subject, through the use of a long-term integrated store, transforms the information from the standard into the modality required for reproduction. He then stores this resulting transformation into short-term memory. It is this memory state, according to Connolly and Jones, which causes the two intermodal conditions to be differentiated. In the kinesthetic-to-visual condition the resulting transformation is stored in visual short-term memory which has characteristics already alluded to in the description of Posner's (1967) work. Information is stored in the form of an image and as long as central processing capacity is available the image can be maintained and reproduced when required. In the other intermodal condition, however, the final transformation is kinesthetic in form and as a consequence it is stored in kinesthetic short-term memory. Again, Connolly and Jones refer to the Posner study (1967) when describing this memory system. According to them it is an unstable memory in that it does not have access to the central processing system and as a result information spontaneously decays. It is this inherent instability of kinesthetic short-term memory that accounts for why the visual-to-kinesthetic condition resulted in relatively inaccurate performance.

There is, however, an alternate explanation to account for the asymmetry between Connolly and Jones' two intermodal matching conditions. It may be that the translation of kinesthetic information into a visual code is more direct and natural than the reverse process and hence asymmetry would be caused by a difference in the translation or coding process rather than by differences in the two memory systems. Further research that differentiates the translation process from the memory process is thus needed before any concrete conclusions can be made.

The other significant feature of the Connolly and Jones' model that is germane to the development of this chapter concerns their concept of the development of the long-term integrated store. It is initially formed by visual and kinesthetic inputs occurring simultaneously with the two streams of information being collated or equated and then stored. Over time a comprehensive store of equated information is built up which can then act to recode visual information into kinesthetic information or vice versa. Changes to the integrated store can come about when an individual detects a mismatch between vision and kinesthesis. He then calculates a new function between the two types of information and stores the end result in the integrated store.

In terms of the purpose of this chapter, the main implication to be derived from the above discussion on the relationship between vision and kinesthesis is that it appears that vision plays a prominent role in the retention of movement information. This role is one of recoding kinesthetic information. In other words, one can think of vision as the basic code by which kinesthetic information is stored in memory and it would be predicted from this that kinesthetic information which is unable to be recoded visually would be subject to spontaneous forgetting. Again, as mentioned previously, this recoding viewpoint may explain the differences between the retention of location and distance cues cited earlier. Furthermore, the question raised at this point is whether kinesthesis can only be recoded into visual form or whether there may be other viable codes. In the nonmotor literature there appears to be a great deal of flexibility as to how information is coded. Certainly, vision would seem to be a dominant code but perhaps other codes like counting or timing (Laabs, 1973) and audition might be used in certain circumstances.

By way of summary, then, it has been established that there are a number of different movement cues that are somehow coded and retained to serve as the internal representation of physical movement. Just how these movement cues are coded is subject to more research but it appears that recoding movement information into a visual form is at least one distinct possibility. Further, the results of some studies indicate that movement information unable to be recoded decays spontaneously and resembles, except in its temporal characteristics, the short-term sensory storage for sense modalities like vision and audition. Evidence was also presented which suggested that the basis of short-term memory for movement information is an integrated sensory store built up through an individual's past experience. Learning of perceptual motor skills would not only depend on modifying this integrated store but also using it to recode relevant movement information about a new task.

III. Movement Production: The Motor Schema

While the above notion of using an integrated store of information to recode movement information can be used to understand the characteristics of motor short-term memory, an integrated store concept can also be utilized to explain how movement information is stored for the production of movement (i.e., motor long-term memory). An example of a type of integrated store used for this purpose has been incorporated into the learning and performance model of Laszlo and Bairstow (1971). The model is composed of a standard, which is the idea or executive program of a given skill that incorporates all the relevant information about the skill, and a motor programming unit which is responsible for assembling a sequence of motor commands for the purpose of executing a movement. The efficiency with which the motor programming unit can assemble appropriate motor commands is dependent on the amount of information contained in the standard. The learner develops this standard through instructions and situational cues, knowledge of results, and sensory feedback from kinesthesis, touch, vision, and audition, as well as feedback from efference. This standard is not only important for storing information about the skill but is also important for controlling movement while actually executing the skill.

According to the model movement control is achieved through a closed-loop system by comparing sensory feedback and efference copy with the standard. It is important to note, however, that while these types of feedback are important for control purposes, according to the model they also have important roles in the learning of movement since they are used to modify the standard. Modification of the standard leads to a more well-defined idea of the movement which in turn leads to a more efficient operation of the motor programming unit.

The main point in presenting this model is to demonstrate how the standard, which could be thought of as an integrated store of movement information, is incorporated into a broader perspective of motor learning and performance. While Laszlo and Bairstow do not stipulate how all the movement information that comprises the standard is coded and organized, they definitely do recognize that a learner of a perceptual-motor skill has various sources of information by which to develop an idea or standard of the skill.

I would like to think that the concept of the standard of movement is rooted in the early thoughts and ideas of Bartlett (1961), who first popularized the concept of the schema. While remaining dormant for several decades this concept is posited as a mechanism in recent analysis of human learning (Pew, 1974; Schmidt, 1975) where the schema plays a central role in describing human perceptual-motor performance. Pew sees the schema, which is roughly equivalent to the idea of the standard as presented in Laszlo and Bairstow's model, as defining the general characteristics about the movement that must be organized to meet specific environmental demands as well as the goal of the performer. Pew believes that the schema represents properties of movement sequences, like spatial patterns, that are encoded and are applicable to a rather large range of specific movements with respect to a particular goal. The exact nature of a specific movement is determined by a schema instance selector which selects the movement in light of the environmental demands and the goal of the performer.

Thus the concept of the schema implies that there is an integrated and generalized store of knowledge about a skill that can be utilized to produce a wide range of unique movements that match specific environmental demands. A good example of the role the schema plays in movement organization is when an individual writes his name by holding the pen in his preferred hand as compared to when he holds it between his teeth. Even though he has probably never attempted the latter skill the generalized spatial patterns representing the movement sequences of his signature, contained within the schema, can be used to reproduce a signature that, although rather shaky, will have a movement pattern similar to the one produced by the hand. There are other obvious examples that illustrate the same point. The football quarterback, in order to be an accurate and consistent passer, must modify his passes to take into account the distance, velocity, and movement patterns of the receiver, wind and other weather conditions, as well as the particular defensive pattern he is faced with. Obviously this requires subtle modification of the movement pattern in the overarm throwing action for each specific situation. What is needed for this translation is a motor schema which, through learning, comes to contain all the generalized integrated parameters that are needed to generate a unique movement to each situation.

Perhaps Bartlett (1961) best described the concept of a schema when he was forming the basis of a theory of remembering. His description and definition of the schema was:

> ... an active organization of past reactions, or of past experiences, which must always be supposed to be operating in any well-adapted organic response. That is, whenever there is any order or regularity of behavior, a particular response is possible only because it is related to other responses which have been serially organized, yet which operate, not simply as individual members coming one after another, but as a unitary mass. Determination by schemata is the most fundamental of all the ways in which we can be influenced by reactions and experiences which occurred some time in the past. All incoming impulses of a certain kind, or mode, go together to build up an active, organized setting: visual, auditory, various types of cutaneous impulses and the like, at a relatively low level; all the experiences connected by a common interest: in sport, in literature, history, art, science, philosophy, and so on, on a higher level. There is not the slightest reason, however, to suppose that each set of incoming impulses, each new group of experiences persists as an isolated member of some passive patchwork. They have to be regarded as constituents of living, momentary settings belonging to the organisms, or to whatever parts of the organism are concerned in making a response of a given kind, and not as a number of individual events somehow strung together and stored within the organism [Bartlett, 1961, Chapter 19, p. 201].

Bartlett stresses the point that memory must not be thought of as reduplicative or reproductive in nature. To support this viewpoint he gives an example of a tennis player making a stroke during a game. The tennis player never just reproduces something he has learned in the past, nor does he produce something new, but rather the stroke is produced by considering the exact nature of the stroke required and then producing a movement that will meet these demands. Thus the memory for movement is constructive in nature, where an individual's past experiences enable him to produce movements that, for any given skill like a stroke in tennis, are never quite the same from time to time but are altered just enough to meet the specific needs of the situation. In this respect, Bartlett's notion of memory as a constructive process is similar to Pew's (1974) concepts of a schema and schema instance. The schema instance is a unique sequence of motor commands manufactured from a rich store of past movement experiences and designed to produce a movement that will meet a specific environmental demand.

Movement memory from the above viewpoint is cognitive in that what is stored are rules or principles that can be applied to a wide range of movements. Hebb (1949) postulated that through learning the perceptual information about a skill becomes internalized so that a skilled individual intellectualizes the skill and uses this cognitive process, in conjunction with feedback from a movement, to control the achievement of any specific environmental demand. According to Hebb the internalization of a skill, which he calls motor equivalence, initially depends on the simultaneous occurrence of perceptual information about the goal of the motor behavior and the particular sensory consequences of the motor activity that an individual employs to achieve the goal.

Lashley (1951), in attempting to explain the same type of intellectualization process for movement production, postulated the existence of "space coordinate systems" that control movement. Here, movement production and control are seen to depend upon internalized spatial representation of the axes of the body and of gravity as well as the space coordinate systems of the environment derived primarily from vision, audition, and touch. This integrated knowledge of the body and environment, gained through experience, can be used to specify the parameters of a movement that will exactly match the environmental demands of a particular situation.

IV. Coding of Movement Information: A Two-Stage Process

To this point, the preceding discussion has established three concepts that are critical when considering the information processes responsible for transforming movement related input information into internal representations of movement: (a) a number of movement-related cues that are important in movement reproduction such as location and distance information (spatial information), counting, and visual information; (b) a visual-kinesthetic integrated store has an important recoding function for movement information, especially for the spatial type; and (c) the motor schema, similar to an integrated store, seems to lie at the base of movement production and hence is intrinsically tied to any discussion of motor memory.

When considering these three points with a human memory system in general one must assume that there is a hierarchy of organization within such a system. For our purpose the most highly organized aspect of motor memory would be the motor schema which is an overall impression or abstract of the parameters influencing movement production. In other words it is both generalized and nonspecific and thus would apply to a wide variety of movement. In terms of what mechanisms underlie this abstraction process and the form of representation the schema takes we are almost totally ignorant. Brooks and Stoney (1971), from neurophysiological evidence, indicate that there are at least three movement control systems: force, velocity, and displacement. Subjectively, one would think that sequential timing (i.e., timing of sequential force commands) would have to be another component of the motor schema.

At a level of organization under that of the schema, however, are information processes that are more directly related to the sensory world and that deal specifically with the coding of sensory information that a performer receives while attempting a movement. At the base of these processes is the notion of an integrated store of movement information similar in form to the integrated store put forward in Connolly and Jones's (1970) model. In essence, however, it is postulated that there are a number of integrated stores dealing with the integration of information from such sources as, for example, vision and kinesthesis, audition and kinesthesis, efference and vision, and timing (counting) and kinesthesis. These integrated stores serve to code sensory information that is relevant to movement and thus represent the first information processing stage in the transformation of input information to some internal representation. In other words, it is postulated that this initial coding process is synonomous with motor short-term memory.

As mentioned above the final form that movement information takes in the motor schema is unknown. The motor schema, however, may be some higher order of integrated information formed from integration of the multiple codes established in motor short-term memory. It would seem, moreover, that the form of information in the motor schema would be unlike that of short-term memory where the code is a relatively direct representation of the sensory world. Rather, the motor schema would most likely be abstractions of these codes from which rules of movement can be formed for the purpose of generating motor commands.

From this viewpoint, then, the transformation of movement information into a permanent internalized form is seen as a two-stage process. First, incoming sensory information is coded by an appropriately developed long-term integrated store that results in a temporary code being stored in motor short-term memory. Since there are opportunities for the development of several integrated stores, motor short-term memory is seen as containing multiple codes of movement information. The second stage in the transformation process concerns the development of the motor schema. Here, codes from motor short-term memory are seen as being integrated and abstracted so that the final form of movement information is analogous to an intellectual process capable of producing a wide range of movements.

References

Adams, J.A., and Dijkstra, S. (1966). *J. Exp. Psychol.* 71, 314–318.
Bartlett, F.C. (1961). "Remembering: A Study in Experimental and Social Psychology." Cambridge Univ. Press, London and New York.

Bilodeau, E.A., Sulzer, J.L., and Levy, C.M. (1962). *Psychol. Monogr.* **76**, No. 20 (Whole No. 539).

Broadbent, D.E. (1971). *Brit. Med. Bull.* **27**, 191–194.

Brooks, J.B., and Stoney, S.D. (1971). *Annu. Rev. Physiol.* **33**, 337–392.

Connolly, K., and Jones, B. (1970). *Brit. J. Psychol.* **61**, 259–266.

Hebb, D.O. (1949). The Organization of Behavior: A Neuropsychological Theory." Wiley, New York.

Jones, B. (1974). *J. Exp. Psychol.* **102**, 37–43.

Keele, S.W. (1973). "Attention and Human Performance." Goodyear, Pacific Palisades, California.

Laabs, G.J. (1973). *J. Exp. Psychol.* **100**, 168–177.

Lashley, K.S. (1917). *Amer. J. Physiol.* **43**, 169–194.

Lashley, K.S. (1951). *In* "Cerebral Mechanisms in Behavior" (L.A. Jeffries, ed.), pp. 112–136. Wiley, New York.

Laszlo, J.I., and Bairstow, P.J. (1971). *J. Mot. Behav.* **3**, 241–252.

Marteniuk, R.G. (1973). *J. Mot. Behav.* **5**, 249–259.

Pew, R.W. (1974). *In* "Human Information Processing: Tutorials in Performance and Cognition" (B.J. Kantowitz, ed.), p. 1. Erlbaum, New York.

Posner, M.I. (1967). *J. Exp. Psychol.* **75**, 103–107.

Posner, M.I. (1969). *In* "Information-Processing Approaches to Visual Perception" (R.N. Haber, ed.), pp. 49–60. Holt, New York.

Schmidt, R.A. (1975). *Psychol. Rev.* **82**, 225–260.

Proprioception as a Basis
of Anticipatory Timing Behavior

Robert W. Christina

I. Introduction

The focus of this chapter is on proprioception as a mechanism underlying the anticipatory timing of movement responses in perceptual anticipation situations. The term proprioception, according to Sherrington (1906), includes sensory information arising from the kinesthetic and the vestibular receptors. He defined proprioception as the sensing of force and extent of movement, muscular tensions, physical pressures, and the position of the body and its parts in space. Anticipatory timing refers to the timing of the overall response relative to some environmental stimulus event. It involves the initiation of an accurate movement response before the actual occurrence of the environmental stimulus event. If the initiation is correct, the resulting effect is a timed response, that is, a response which occurs simultaneously or in close time coincidence with the occurrence of the stimulus event.

One means by which a subject makes timed responses is anticipation. It allows the subject to prepare his movement responses in advance of stimulus event occurrences so that they can be made in the "right" place at the "right" time in relation to these occurrences. Although several types of anticipation have been conceptualized (Bartlett, 1951; Belisle, 1963; Poulton, 1957a), the present chapter is concerned with the type referred to as perceptual anticipation; it operates in situations where the subject receives no preview or advance information about the forthcoming stimulus events to which he must respond. Adams (1966) identifies two types of perceptual anticipation: spatial and temporal. Spatial anticipation requires that the subject predict where a stimulus event will appear, while temporal anticipation demands that he predict when it will appear. The perceptual anticipation of motor responses requires that the subject be able to predict the nature and size of his muscular contractions as well as the direction, extent, and duration of his movement so that it can be made properly in relation to environmental stimulus events. In order to predict accurately, the subject must learn the pattern of regularities in the forthcoming stimulus events so that with repeated event occurrences he can retrieve the pattern information from long-term memory and use it as a rule to prepare his movement response before the stimulus event arrives at some future position. Evidence from tracking studies (Noble and Trumbo, 1967; Poulton, 1952a,b, 1957b) indicate that early in learning the responses are guided by environmental stimuli and that later in learning there is less dependence on the environmental stimuli because the cues for responding have become internalized. Once the cues are internalized the subject can rely on his memory of the environmental stimuli to prepare for the time when movement responses are to be made.

A central question for understanding anticipatory timing performance in perceptual anticipation situations is the means by which the subject can judge the duration prior to a stimulus occurrence so as to effectively anticipate. Many mechanisms have been proposed to explain how a subject keeps time. However, a close examination of the many different mechanisms reveals that most of them hypothesize some sort of "time base" which is believed to generate cues at successive points in time (Michon, 1967). Although the notion of a basic unit of subjective time is fundamental to the "time base" concept, unequivocal evidence for a universal time quantum has not been found.

Perhaps this failure to find a universal time quantum is one reason why other explanations, such as Ornstein's (1969) information-processing theory, have been proposed. Ornstein's theory attempts to account for the effect of stimulus complexity on time perception and essentially it holds that time-keeping is a mental construction, resulting directly from the subject's perception of the particular physical characteristics of the stimulus events defining a given interval.

Ornstein's theory is consistent with Yeager's (1969) ideas and has received some recent support from Schiffman and Bobko (1974). The theory seems to be a viable explanation of time-keeping, but more research is needed before its validity can be ascertained in relation to motor tasks.

In situations involving motor tasks, it has been hypothesized that proprioception can serve as one possible time-keeping mechanism in the accurate anticipatory timing of movement responses (Adams and Creamer, 1962a,b; Schmidt, 1968, 1971; Schmidt and Christina, 1969). Essentially, two views have emerged which describe how the proprioceptive mechanism operates. One view is referred to as the proprioceptive trace hypothesis and the other is called the proprioceptive input hypothesis. Although both hypotheses are in agreement that propriocetion can serve as a time-keeping mechanism, there is a difference of opinion as to how the proprioceptive stimuli are used. The present chapter will describe these two hypotheses and critically review the evidence offered as support for them. In addition, alternative explanations involving "motor outflow" and the "preprogramming" of motor responses as a basis for anticipatory timing will be discussed.

II. Proprioceptive Trace Hypothesis

The proprioceptive trace hypothesis was originally discussed by Adams and Xhignesse (1960), Adams (1961), and Adams and Creamer (1962a) to account for the anticipatory timing of movement responses in perceptual anticipation situations. The hypothesis was formally stated by Adams and Creamer (1962b) and it proposes that

> . . . the time-persisting proprioceptive after-effects of an overt or mediated response can be the mechanism to account for motor timing behavior. The occurrence of a response at time t is assumed to generate a time-varying stimulus trace, and the stimulus characteristics of the trace at time $t + \Delta t$ is the cue set to which the subject learns the response that is anticipatory to the environmental event by being initiated without a specific environmental cue.

Essentially, the trace hypothesis is a stimulus-response (S-R) view which assumes that movements can be conditioned to traces of proprioceptive stimulus aftereffects and that, with practice, the occurrence of a correct pattern of stimulus aftereffects can elicit the next correct movement sequence.

A. Original Evidence for the Trace Hypothesis

When Adams and Creamer (1962a) found that mediational responses acquired through pretraining transferred positively to anticipatory timing of arm-hand movements in the whole pursuit tracking task, they proposed the trace hypothesis as one possible explanation. Pretraining neutral responses consisted of saying the word "change," pressing a button, or moving a small crank handle over a 180° distance in response to the directional change of a sine-wave input requiring perceptual anticipation. The same sine-wave input was used in the whole task. Evidence for mediation as a mechanism for anticipatory timing seemed to be found when all three pretraining responses transferred positively to the timing of movements in the whole task. Assuming an S-R position, Adams and Creamer discussed the possibility that proprioceptive stimulation was the common element associated with all these mediating responses. Proprioceptive traces from persisting fractional movements related to these responses may have formed the mediational basis for anticipatory timing. Consequently, they hypothesized that the aftereffects of a movement response (pretraining response) made earlier in time (at time t) persist, and provide internal cues to which the criterion movement response is learned for anticipatory occurrence at a later time (time $t + \Delta t$).

The Adams and Creamer (1962a) results can also be explained from a cognitive position. It can be argued that all three pretraining methods allowed the subject to visually perceive the time patterning of stimulus events which was sufficient for acquiring anticipatory timing in the whole task. On the other hand, if there is any validity to the trace hypothesis, anticipatory timing in tracking should emerge as some function of the task variables (e.g., spring loading) that are assumed to define levels of proprioception (Bahrick, 1957), since higher levels should provide more distinct proprioceptive aftereffects than lower levels. In addition, timing should also emerge as some function of the time between responses on the basis that the trace is decaying over time and has a more efficacious cuing character at a shorter duration than a longer one.

Adams and Creamer (1962b) tested these ideas in an experiment in which there were two levels of spring loading (no spring loading or spring loading), two amplitudes of movement (2¾ in. or 7¾ in.), and two stimulus event durations (2 or 4 sec). A one-dimensional, discrete visual-tracking task was used in which subjects had to learn to anticipate and time the initiation of horizontal arm movements to repetitive and regular, step-input signal changes of either 2 or 4 sec. The results indicated that the shorter duration between responses provided for more proficient anticipatory timing than the longer duration. Although amplitude of movement was not a significant contributor to anticipatory timing, spring loading was and better timing resulted from moving the spring loaded control than from moving the unloaded control. Despite the failure for the amplitude factor, Adams and Creamer proposed that these results not only strengthened the mediational explanation of the trace hypothesis proposed in their previous study (Adams and Creamer, 1962a), but also confirmed the hypothesis with regard to overt instrumental responses.

B. Limitations of the Original Evidence and
Further Research

Although the trace hypothesis appears to have been supported, there are two methodological problems with the Adams and Creamer study (1962b) that warrant some discussion. First, in order to determine that it was the decay of proprioceptive aftereffects which the subject was using to cue the timing of his next response, it must be shown that he was not simultaneously receiving cues from any other source after the movement. However, subjects in the spring-loaded condition had to voluntarily contract the appropriate muscles in such a way that the resistance of the control could be overcome so that the control could be held on target in a stationary position. In this situation, the subject could have been receiving cues from the proprioceptive stimulation generated by the muscular contractions needed to hold the control in a stationary position or from the efference required to effect those contractions. Second, spring loading was manipulated on the same limb that was used to effect the timed responses and it is possible that the spring-loaded responses were facilitated more than the unloaded responses not because the former condition produced a higher level of proprioceptive aftereffects, but because it resulted in a more favorable mechanical system for responding. Thus, the effects due to proprioception and the mechanics of the response control system were confounded.

Christina (1970) attempted to avoid the methodological problems of the Adams and Creamer study (1962b) and subject the trace hypothesis to another test. He indirectly varied levels of proprioception by manipulating load and amplitude of movement on a control operated by a limb (left arm) different than the one (right arm) which was used to effect the timed finger response. Experimental conditions included no movement, unloaded movement, and loaded movement which were assumed to generate minimum moderate, and maximum levels of proprioceptive cues, respectively. The subjects could not view their left-arm movement at any time. The movement part of the task required each subject in the left-arm movement conditions to voluntarily move a control linearly 13 in. along a track; when the end of the track was reached, he was to rest his limb on an armrest in a stationary position. This resting stationary position should have allowed the aftereffects generated from the left-arm movement to decay during the interval (2 sec) between the end of the movement and the occurrence of the environmental stimulus event. The timing task required the subject to learn to use the appropriate stimulus configuration of the aftereffects to cue the right-finger response so that it would occur coincidentally with the stimulus event. If the trace hypothesis was operating, higher levels of proprioceptive aftereffects should facilitate response timing more than lower levels. The results were negative and failed to support the trace hypothesis.

Quesada and Schmidt (1970) suggested that failure to support the trace hypothesis in the Christina study was due to the fact that the left-arm movements were not consistent enough from trial to trial. If these movements were excessively variable, it is likely that their traces of aftereffects were variable also, thus not giving the subject an adequate opportunity to condition his movements to those traces. In an attempt to resolve this consistency problem Quesada and Schmidt used a passive, motor-driven, left-arm movement. Experimental conditions consisted of no left-arm movement and passive left-arm movement. The movement part of the task required each subject in the movement condition to grasp a control located above his head with his left hand and hold on while his left arm was moved passively downward along a track 26 in. in length. When the limb reached the end of the track it was rested on the arm of a chair in a stationary position to permit the aftereffects produced from the movement to decay during the interval (2 sec) between the end of the movement and the occurrence of an environmental stimulus event. The timing task required that the subject learn to use the appropriate stimulus pattern of aftereffects to cue the right-finger response so that it would occur simultaneously with the stimulus event. The results indicated that subjects with movement had less absolute error, constant error, and variable error than the subjects without movement. These results were viewed as support for the trace hypothesis, and indicated that Christina (1970) may not have found supporting evidence because of the inconsistency of his subject's left-arm movements.

C. Summary

The study by Adams and Creamer (1962b) did not provide evidence which clearly supported the trace hypothesis. This was the case because either proprioception or efference itself may have served as cues during the interval between movements and because the effects due to proprioception and the mechanics of the responding system were confounded. Christina (1970) attempted to untangle these confounding elements, but his results were negative. However, Quesada and Schmidt (1970) recognized the left-arm movement consistency problem in the Christina study and controlled for this variability in their experiment by using a motor-driven passive movement. Their results supported the trace hypothesis and this appears to be the only source of evidence that clearly does so.

III. Proprioceptive Input Hypothesis

The possibility of proprioceptive cues operating during the interval between movements in the Adams and Creamer experiment (1962b) and the preliminary evidence (Ellis, 1969; Ellis *et al.*, 1968; Goldfarb and Goldstone, 1963; Goldstone *et al.*, 1958) which indicates that movement made during an interval to be judged enhances the accuracy of estimating the duration of that interval, prompted Schmidt and Christina (1969) to offer a different explanation than the one proposed by the trace hypothesis. Their explanation is referred to as the input hypothesis and it proposes that incoming proprioceptive feedback, produced by movement made during the interval preceding the occurrence of a stimulus event, is the means by which a subject judges the duration of the interval so as to accurately anticipate the stimulus occurrence. It is assumed that the subject comes to use the incoming proprioceptive feedback through learning, but exactly how the feedback mechanism operates is not understood. Schmidt (1971) proposed one explanation which holds that the pattern of proprioceptive feedback produced from the earlier portion of a movement response can function to cue a later portion. Presumably, the proprioceptive feedback possesses stimulus characteristics and the subject learns the specific characteristics which will cue the later portion of the response that is supposed to occur simultaneously with the environmental stimulus event. However, there is no evidence presently which clearly indicates that the mechanism operates as Schmidt has suggested.

A. Preliminary Evidence Leading to the Input Hypothesis

The studies which follow prompted the formulation of the input hypothesis. Essentially these studies provide evidence that movement-filled intervals are timed more accurately than unfilled ones. Further, they hypothesize that proprioception can serve as a time perception mechanism.

Goldstone *et al.* (1958) had subjects estimate a 1-sec interval by counting aloud and to oneself for 30.0 sec at a rate of 1 count/sec. Foot and finger tapping were permitted when counting aloud, but not when counting to oneself (restricted condition). The results indicated that counting aloud and tapping produced more accurate estimates than the restricted condition. They hypothesized that counting aloud and tapping produced more proprioceptive cues and a better basis for estimating time than the restricted condition. Further investigation by Goldfarb and Goldstone (1963) revealed that either overt counting or small manipulatory movements made during the interval (1 sec) to be judged produced more accurate estimates than when no verbal counting or observable movement was available during the interval. They also hypothesized that proprioception was the basis for the more accurate time estimates.

Ellis *et al.* (1968) used an operative estimation task in which subjects had to estimate 2 sec by moving a control along a track. Amplitude of movement was manipulated so that the distance moved during the interval was either 2.5 or 65.0 cm. Load on the control was also varied so that movement was made with either no load or an 8.5 lb load. The results indicated that the 65.0-cm movement resulted in more accurate absolute error estimates later in practice than the 2.5-cm movement. No significant load effects were found, but on the basis of the movement effects they hypothesized that the larger movement produced a greater amount of proprioceptive cues and a more effective basis for estimating time than the smaller movement.

Employing an operative estimation task similar to Ellis *et al.* (1968), Ellis (1969) attempted to demonstrate that the accuracy of judging time depended on proprioceptive feedback produced during the interval (2.0 sec) to be estimated. He manipulated acceleration cues by varying the inertia of the control system, velocity cues by varying the viscous resistance of the control, and tension cues by varying spring loading on the control. The results revealed that resistance proportional to the velocity and acceleration produced more accurate and consistent absolute error estimates in fewer trials than an unresisted movement. Tension proportional to position failed to have a significant effect on operative estimation performance. Ellis also had subjects spell a random arrangement of 2-, 3- and 4-letter words at conversational level while auditory cues from spelling were masked by simulated white noise. He found that spelling 3- and 4-letter words produced more accurate estimates than spelling 2-letter words or no words at all. Ellis generally concluded that the greater proprioceptive feedback cues produced from resistance proportional to velocity and acceleration and from spelling 3- and 4-letter words provides a better basis for estimating time than unresisted or minimal-movement conditions.

B. Limitations of the Preliminary Evidence and Further Research

One limitation of the studies by Goldstone *et al.* (1958) and Goldfarb and Goldstone (1963) was that auditory cues associated with the manipulatory movements and counting aloud were permitted to operate in the movement-filled interval, but not in the unfilled interval. Thus, effects due to the auditory cues and the movement cues were confounded. A limitation common to studies by Ellis *et al.* (1968) and Ellis (1969) was that task variables defining levels of proprioception were manipulated in the same limb that was used for the operative estimation response. It is possible that manipulating feedback in the responding limb enhances estimates simply because it creates a more favorable mechanical system for responding. Thus, it seems that the spelling effect found by Ellis (1969) was the only source of preliminary evidence which was not confounded with auditory or mechanical effects.

In an attempt to avoid these limitations, Schmidt and Christina (1969) masked auditory cues with simulated white noise and indirectly varied levels of proprioceptive feedback by manipulating amplitude of movement on a control operated by a limb (left arm) that was different than the one (right arm) which was used to effect the timed finger response. Experimental conditions included a minimal 0.5-in. movement, moderate movement through a 3.5-in. radius of rotation, and large movement through a 11.5-in. radius of rotation which were assumed to generate minimal, intermediate, and high levels of proprioceptive cues, respectively. The task required each subject in the movement conditions to voluntarily rotate a crank handle with the left arm while the timing response was effected with the right finger. The timing response required that the subject release his finger from a response key simultaneously with the occurrence of an environmental stimulus event. Based on the assumption that the level of proprioceptive feedback was related to the size of the left-arm movement, it was hypothesized that the larger the left-arm movement the more effective the basis for judging duration and timing the response of the right finger. Support for the hypothesis was found when the moderate-sized rotary movement resulted in significantly more "beneficial anticipations" (percentage of responses which occurred within 133 msec of the stimulus event) than the minimal-movement condition. However, this finding did not completely support the hypothesis since large-sized rotary movement did not result in significantly more "beneficial anticipations" than the moderate movement. Further investigation revealed that the large movement was more inconsistent from trial to trial than the moderate movement. It was hypothesized that the inconsistency of the large movement provided a more variable pattern of proprioceptive cues and a poorer basis for timing the right-finger response than the moderate movement.

Schmidt and Christina also computed within-subject correlation coefficients between the extent of the left-arm movement on a given trial and the constant error of the right-finger response on that trial for each subject separately. The results indicated that at least half the subjects tended to covary the extent of the left-arm movement with the error of the right-finger response. It was further hypothesized that those subjects with high correlations were relying on proprioceptive feedback of the position of their movement to cue the timing of the right-finger response.

Christina also investigated the input hypothesis by using the procedure developed by Schmidt and Christina (1969) which consisted of manipulating movement or task variables (e.g., load) in the left arm while the timing response is effected by the right-index finger. In the first study, Christina (1970) found that subjects with movement performed the timing response with less variable error than subjects without movement. In addition, he found that about half the subjects covaried their left-arm movement velocities with the constant error of their right-finger response. The second study (Christina, 1971) differed from previous research (Christina, 1970; Schmidt and Christina, 1969) in that the subjects in the second study were explicitly instructed to use their left-arm movement to time their right-finger response. The results revealed that subjects with movement performed the timing response with less absolute error than subjects without movement. Further, he found that about 94% of the subjects covaried the extent of their left-arm movement with the constant error of their right-finger response.

C. Summary

Some of the preliminary evidence which seems to be consistent with the input hypothesis must be approached with caution since two of these studies (Gold-stone *et al.*, 1958; Goldfarb and Goldstone, 1963) confounded auditory and movement effects and two others (Ellis *et al.*, 1968; Ellis, 1969) confounded mechanical and proprioceptive effects. However, the spelling effect found by Ellis (1969), and the movement effects of Schmidt and Christina (1969) and Christina (1970, 1971) are free of such confounding and they are sources of evidence which clearly indicates that voluntary movement during the interval to be judged facilitates the proficiency of estimating the duration of that interval. But there is no conclusive evidence to indicate that the proficiency of judging duration varies directly with the level of force requirements or amount of movement during the interval. Further, although all the studies reviewed in Section III hypothesize a connection between proprioception and anticipatory timing, there is no convincing evidence that incoming proprioceptive feedback, produced by movement made during the interval, is the means by which a subject judges the duration of the interval so as to accurately anticipate the stimulus occurrences. Thus, the validity of the input hypothesis has yet to be determined.

IV. Issues and Trends

A. Proprioceptive Trace Hypothesis

Presently, there is only one source of evidence (Quesada and Schmidt, 1970) clearly supporting the trace hypothesis. However, that evidence is limited to a situation involving passive left-arm movements and the anticipatory timing of a motor response in a discrete task. The hypothesis needs to be tested using voluntary movements, but avoiding the confounding variables which plagued earlier studies (Adams and Creamer, 1962b; Christina, 1970). Research investigating the validity of the hypothesis with regard to anticipatory timing of motor responses in seria' and continuous tasks is also needed. Further, the hypothesis must be tested for mediational responses as well as for overt instrumental responses. If the hypothesis withstands these preliminary empirical tests, more faith can be placed in time-varying proprioceptive traces as one possible time-perception mechanism in the accurate anticipatory timing of motor responses.

B. Proprioceptive Input Hypothesis

The evidence (Christina, 1970, 1971; Ellis, 1969; Schmidt and Christina, 1969) supporting the input hypothesis may not be as convincing as it seems since there is no conclusive evidence that proprioceptive feedback actually functioned as basis for anticipatory timing. Further, the spelling and the left-arm movements were voluntary actions which involved the outflow of efferent signals from the central nervous system to the appropriate muscles and subjects may have been using the outflow as a basis for timing their responses (Jones, 1973, 1974; Schmidt, 1973). Essentially, the outflow view holds that the timing of movements are preprogrammed by means of some internalized "image of efference" or an "efference copy" (von Holst, 1954). Jones (1974) has proposed that the temporal order of the sequence of efferent commands needed to effect movements appropriately may be controlled by the circulation of the "image" between the motor cortex and the cerebellum. If Jones is correct, it is possible for the "image" itself to provide the basis for timing future efferent signals without the use of proprioceptive or peripheral feedback. For example, in the Schmidt and Christina study (1969), subjects could have preprogrammed the extent of each left-arm movement and cued the timing of the right-finger response on a central rather than on a proprioceptive or peripheral basis.

Resolving this issue will not be an easy task. However, Jones (1973) has suggested that one approach to begin with would be to try to replicate the studies claiming support for the input hypothesis, but to use passive rather than voluntary movements. He encouraged the use of a passive-type movement because there would be no efference or outflow to the limb to effect movement, but there would be proprioceptive inflow from the limb as a result of movement. Whatever approach is used it is obvious that further research is needed before the validity of the input hypothesis or the outflow hypothesis can be determined.

C. Alternative Views

Other explanations of the time-perception mechanism in the anticipatory timing of motor responses are possible. For example, one might hypothesize that the anticipatory timing of highly learned responses in perceptual anticipation situations are completely preprogrammed, that is, independent of any central feedback-loop monitoring of efference as suggested in Section IV,B. The "image of efference" or "motor program" (Keele, 1968) would itself control response timing by running its course in an open-loop manner without modification. In this situation, the "image" would be modified by the occasional monitoring of response outcome information rather than by the central monitoring of efference.

On the basis of a study by Pew (1966), it also seems reasonable to postulate an inflow-outflow compromise explanation which accounts for both sensory feedback (inflow) and central-loop monitoring of efference (outflow). Essentially, the explanation is based on a model proposed by Fitts (1962, 1964) and it holds that with a large amount of practice a master plan is developed within which preprogrammed routines are integrated. The preprogrammed routines would have central feedback loops monitoring efference, while the master plan would monitor the response output information and be modified by sensory feedback. The anticipatory timing of responses would be controlled by the central monitoring of efference of the preprogrammed subroutines comprising the master plan and would not be changed unless the master plan was modified by sensory feedback.

D. Concluding Comments

It is not certain whether the bases of anticipatory timing are a trace of proprioceptive aftereffects, an incoming pattern of proprioceptive feedback, outflow with or without central efferent monitoring, a compromise model consisting of a master plan with preprogrammed routines, or some other mechanism which has not been considered. Perhaps proprioceptive mechanisms have their significance as a state of transition to central outflow mechanisms which come to control anticipatory timing at the advanced stages of skill. There does not appear to be any conclusive evidence that would support this latter notion. Determining the bases of anticipatory timing in perceptual anticipation situations will be a major undertaking. A systematic research effort dealing with the hypotheses discussed in this chapter is needed before we can determine the means by which a subject anticipates stimulus events so as to accurately time his responses with their occurrences.

References

Adams, J.A. (1961). *Psychol. Bull.* **58**, 55–79.
Adams, J.A. (1966). *In* "Acquisition of Skill" (E.A. Bilodeau, ed.), pp. 169–200. Academic Press, New York.
Adams, J.A., and Creamer, L.R. (1962a). *J. Exp. Psychol.* **63**, 84–90.
Adams, J.A., and Creamer, L.R. (1962b). *Hum. Factors* 4, 217–222.
Adams, J.A., and Xhignesse, L.V. (1960). *J. Exp. Psychol.* **60**, 391–403.
Bahrick, H.P. (1957). *Psychol. Rev.* **64**, 324–328.
Bartlett, F.C. (1951). *In* "Essays in Psychology" (G. Ekman *et al.,* eds.), pp. 1–17. Almqvist & Wiksell, Stockholm.
Belisle, J.J. (1963). *Res. Quart.* **34**, 271–281.
Christina, R.W. (1970). *J. Mot. Behav.* **2**, 125–133.
Christina, R.W. (1971). *J. Mot. Behav.* **3**, 97–104.
Ellis, M.J. (1969). *J. Mot. Behav.* **1**, 119–134.
Ellis, M.J., Schmidt, R.A., and Wade, M.G. (1968). *Ergonomics* **11**, 577–586.

Fitts, P.M. (1962). *In* "Training Research and Education" (R. Glaser, ed.), pp. 177–197. Univ. of Pittsburgh Press, Pittsburgh, Pennsylvania.

Fitts, P.M. (1964). *In* "Categories of Human Learning" (A.W. Melton, ed.), pp. 243–285. Academic Press, New York.

Goldfarb, J., and Goldstone, S. (1963). *Percept. Mot. Skills* 17, 286.

Goldstone, S., Boardman, W.K., and Lhamon, W.T. (1958). *Percept. Mot. Skills* 93, 185–190.

Jones, B. (1973). *Psychol. Bull.* 79, 386–388.

Jones, B. (1974). *J. Mot. Behav.* 6, 33–45.

Keele, S.W. (1968). *Psychol. Bull.* 70, 387–403.

Michon, J.A. (1967). "Timing in Temporal Tracking." Institute for Perception, Soesterberg, The Netherlands.

Noble, M., and Trumbo, D. (1967). *Org. Behav. Hum. Performance* 2, 1–35.

Ornstein, R.E. (1969). "On the Experience of Time." Penquin Books, London.

Pew, R.W. (1966). *J. Exp. Psychol.* 71, 764–771.

Poulton, E.C. (1952a). *Brit. J. Psychol.* 43, 222–229.

Poulton, E.C. (1952b). *Brit. J. Psychol.* 43, 295–302.

Poulton, E.C. (1957a). *J. Exp. Psychol.* 54, 28–32.

Poulton, E.C. (1957b). *Psychol. Bull.* 54, 467–478.

Quesada, D.C., and Schmidt, R.A. (1970). *J. Mot. Behav.* 2, 273–283.

Schiffman, H.R., and Bobko, D.J. (1974). *J. Exp. Psychol.* 103, 156–159.

Schmidt, R.A. (1968). *Psychol. Bull.* 70, 631–646.

Schmidt, R.A. (1971). *Psychol.. Bull.* 76, 383–393.

Schmidt, R.A. (1973). *Psychol. Bull.* 79, 389–390.

Schmidt, R.A., and Christina, R.W. (1969). *J. Exp. Psychol.* 81, 303–307.

Sherrington, C.S. (1906). "The Integrative Action of the Nervous System." Scribner's, New York.

von Holst, E. (1954). *Brit. J. Anim. Behav.* 2, 89–94.

Yeager, J. (1969). *Psychonom. Sci.* 15, 177–178.

Dimensions of Motor Task Complexity

Keith C. Hayes
Ronald G. Marteniuk

I. Introduction

The problem of how man organizes and controls his vast repertoire of complex motor skills is indeed a perplexing one and one that has intrigued scholars from many different disciplines. One particularly contentious issue has been that of identifying and defining those ingredients of the perceptual-motor process that constitute the elements of task complexity. On the one hand, it is recognized that any form of movement possesses degrees of complexity in its enactment by the musculoskeletal system. In this case movement complexity can be equated to the degree of structural organization of the effector units within the central nervous system that eventually lead to movement initiation and control. The variables that affect this process may take the form of the number of muscle groups utilized, the precision of the terminal location, or the frequency of a limb's directional changes. On the other hand, movement complexity may be considered in terms of the degree of involvement of a performer's cognitive processes that are concerned with transforming a stimulus, whether it be from the environment or intrinsic feedback from his response, into an appropriate movement. Movement complexity can then be seen as a function of the number, as well as the attention demands, of decisions involved in the perceptual, translation, and effector mechanisms (Welford, 1968) that lead to movement initiation and control. When viewed in this way it becomes apparent that no simple unilateral definition of task complexity is likely to satisfy all conditions.

One convenient way to grasp a fairly wide perspective of task complexity is to view it from two of the principal approaches to understanding motor control. These two approaches, the "preprogramming model" and the "information processing" approach, may be thought of as being different dimensions, each capable of providing insight into the nature of task complexity. The present chapter is thus devoted to a treatment of motor task complexity as viewed from these two perspectives.

II. Motor Programming and Response Complexity

Reviews of the behavioral literature pertaining to motor programming have been provided by Keele (1968, 1973) and more recently by Schmidt (1975). In essence, the notion of motor programming embodies the view that stored sets of motor commands, both innate and learned, are available within the central nervous system to be called upon at will and synthesized into a desired movement. To be consistent with this previous work we will use the term "motor program" to refer to a collection of motor commands which, when sequentially and temporally ordered, produce a given movement. Smaller subgroups of motor commands which represent components of a movement will be referred to as "subroutines." We thus view the motor program as a carefully coordinated sequence of subroutines which together comprise the desired movement and which are not dependent upon feedback.

The above definition of the motor program is not far removed from the original ideas of Lashley (1917), whose work with a patient deprived of sensation led to development of the programming concept. Lashley's patient, who suffered a gunshot wound in the spinal cord, was capable of reproducing active movements in the absence of proprioceptive feedback from the affected limb. Subsequent work by investigators such as Taub (Taub and Berman, 1963; Taub *et al.*, 1965, 1966), Bossom (1974), and Laszlo (1966; Laszlo and Manning, 1970) has added further support to the view that precise motor control and, for that matter, the learning of motor skills are possible for subjects deprived of feedback from their limbs. Observations such as these, when coupled with the finding that movements can be initiated and corrected in less time than is required for a visual RT (Hick, 1949; Higgins and Angel, 1970), have been taken as support for a centrally initiated sequencing of subroutines capable of being timed and ordered independently of feedback.

Motor programming provides the most parsimonious explanation for the control of movements initiated and terminated completely within approximately 0.2 sec (a normal visual RT). Such movements are frequently described as "ballistic" as their kinematics are completely determined by consecutive bursts of activity in the agonist and antagonist muscles. The latter burst of muscle activity, which causes the "braking" action, is initiated so soon following the agonist activity that it would appear to be part of a centrally initiated motor program that controls the total movement independently of feedback.

We maintain that there is sufficient evidence to suggest that motor programming is used as the basis of more than a trivial number of motor activities and, as such, warrants elaboration. Further, an issue that is particularly relevant to the question of motor task complexity is to determine the composition of (a) the subroutines and (b) the motor program. In essence, we view identification of the composition of these two constructs as one approach to understanding task complexity and it is to this issue that we address the balance of discussion in this section.

A. Motor Programs

A view held by Pew (1974) and reiterated by Schmidt is that ". . . the idea of a motor program is largely a default argument" and that there ". . . is really no direct human evidence of a motor program" (Schmidt, 1975). Schmidt goes on to indicate that satisfactory direct evidence would need to show (1) that feedback is present in movement but not used or (2) that feedback is not present and movement can still occur. Because few data of this nature are available, centralists (proponents of motor programming) are viewed as merely accepting motor programs as the explanation for motor phenomena that cannot be explained by closed-loop theory.

It should, perhaps, be recognized that other criteria do exist for "direct human evidence" in support of the idea of motor programs and subroutines. The significance of experimental evidence based upon these other criteria appears, however, to have received only a modicum of attention in earlier reviews of motor programming. One criterion for "direct human evidence" would be the demonstration in man of stereotyped "fragments" of motion that are capable of being concatenated into complex motor patterns, modified according to the "intent" of the subject, and capable of being appropriately conditioned. As Easton (1972) has so carefully elaborated, such fragments do most definitely exist in the human being in the form of inherent reflex patterns. Far from being the inflexible, nonadaptive rigid structures they were once thought, the body's reflex patterns are now viewed, in the light of recent evidence, as being adaptable and susceptible to conditioning. It is to consideration of this hypothesis that the body's reflexes are functionally equivalent to subroutines of the motor program that we now turn.

1. The Reflex Subroutine: A Hypothesis

Easton's treatise (1972) on coordination and, in particular, his elaboration on a hypothesized reflex pattern substrate of voluntary movement provides a logical starting point:

> The basic argument in support of the inference is that of economy: the central nervous system (CNS) is designed to respond automatically to certain stimuli with certain basic reflexes or "coordinative structures" (CS's), a term meaning only that the response involves one or more muscles working together and intended to add to the word "reflex" the hypothetical quality of underlying all volitionally composed movements. Each such response may be activated by a single command, of either peripheral or central origin, and the CNS may be said to have at its disposal a library, or set, of these responses. It would not be economical if this library of prearranged responses, this CS set, were ignored when volitional movements had to be composed. It would be both simpler and faster to choose and concatenate—perhaps orchestrate—elements of the CS set into one grand volitional coordinative structure than to compose such a structure out of individual muscle contractions or changes in joint angles, even though the muscle and limb state data available to the sensorimotor cortex are known to take the forms of tension, length, joint angle changes, and their time derivatives (Granit, 1970). Use of the CS set would involve much less information processing, less work—just as it is easier and faster to build a house from prefabricated components than from raw lumber and nails [Easton, 1972, p. 591].

The coordinative structures, the body's reflexes, are most familiar to clinicians who frequently see them manifest in the normal course of development of the neonate or in the motor expression of the brain-damaged and mentally retarded. Spinal reflexes such as the stretch reflex are readily identified but the higher level reflexes, (e.g., labyrinthine and righting reflexes) are less well known. More surprising is the fact that the motor acts of stepping and grasping, and in certain instances, scratching, hopping, jumping, and shaking all have as a substrate a primitive reflex. In this regard "reflex" is used in its classic sense in that it connotes an automatic and repeatable subconscious motor response to an appropriate stimulus. The point to be made here is that a vast "vocabulary" of reflex patterns exists in normal man and thus could not only serve as subroutines of motor programs but also could provide a very convenient means for minimizing the complexity of the control process.

In much the same way that voluntary movements have been viewed in terms of a hierarchically structured organization (Bryan and Harter, 1899; Welford, 1968) so too may the reflexes. Using Greene's (1971) concept of elemental and tuning inputs, Easton (1972, 1975) has suggested that elemental reflexes (corresponding to gross approximations of portions of a desired movement) may be identified, as well as tuning reflexes necessary for the biasing and fine adjustments of movement.

An important feature of this hypothesis is that the reflex patterns need not necessarily be elicited only by peripheral stimuli. In Figure 1 a double reciprocal

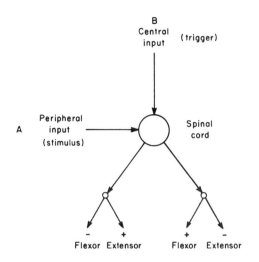

Figure 1 A double reciprocal inhibition schema indicating that the same combination of flexion and extension (a synergy) may be elicited by either an external input (stimulus A) or a centrally triggered input (stimulus B).

inhibition scheme is depicted where the same ipsilateral and contralateral motor effects would be seen whether the stimulus originated peripherally (A), or centrally (B). A reciprocal "synergy,"[1] of this type could thus be triggered by either a centrally initiated command or by peripheral input. Its sustained and smooth operation may, of course, be contingent upon local feedback providing the adequate stimulus for subsequent responses, or alternatively for the modulation of a centrally regulated pattern.

One important implication of the "wired-in" motor pattern represented in Figure 1 is that the response is organized at the level of the spinal cord and that it need only be triggered by the input. This brings to mind the cybernetic principle espoused by Arbib (1972) of distributed motor control processes alleviating any one part of the nervous system of excessive computational demands. In the present context this implies that a subroutine of a motor act (e.g., the stepping reflex or synergy) may be physically located far from the central processor, the brain, and may thus relieve the main program of many burdensome computational details required for specifying limb interactions. Welford (1968) has presented arguments for the organization of voluntary movement along identical lines of reasoning.

Although the case represented in Figure 1 is a simplistic one it serves to

---

[1] The term "synergy" has developed in the Russian literature (e.g., Kots, 1969; Pal'tsev, 1967) to indicate subclasses, or subsets, of movements and may be regarded as being essentially the same as subroutines or reflexes (Easton, 1975).

illustrate the possible use of wired-in reflex patterns as subroutines in a motor program and the idea of distributed motor-control processes. It is appropriate at this point to emphasize that in normal healthy man a vast array of reflex patterns are inherent within the central nervous system. Furthermore, when attempts have been made to analyze normal human motor behavior from the perspective of identifying the reflex patterns in voluntary expression, results have been encouraging. For example, Fukuda (1961), in Japan, has identified the contribution of tonic neck and labyrinthine reflexes in activities including tennis, baseball, judo, and soccer. Although viewed from a different perspective, a number of other studies also provide supportive evidence (Gardner, 1968; Hellebrandt et al., 1956, 1962; O'Connell and Gardner, 1972; Twitchell, 1970).

Perhaps the greatest contributions to the idea of centrally initiated subroutines for movement have come from the study of locomotion. Extensive work by Soviet (Shik et al., 1966; Orlovsky, 1972) and Western investigators (see, for example, Kennedy, 1973) has developed beyond much doubt that, in cats and dogs, locomotor subroutines are evident at segmental levels. Represented in Figure 2 is a speculative scheme of the circuitry involved in the generation of locomotion. This scheme, taken from the work of Grillner (1973), indicates that the "step generator," the locomotor subroutine, does not act autonomously but is influenced by unspecified inputs which serve to intensify the general excitability level. The step generator, which involves spinal interneurons, and may involve a synthesis of a number of spinal reflex patterns, is brought into action by one or more of the descending supraspinal systems. The descending reticulo-spinal noradrenergic fibers are prime candidates for this role. Also, spinal inputs may, under certain circumstances, serve to release the interneuronal stepping generator.

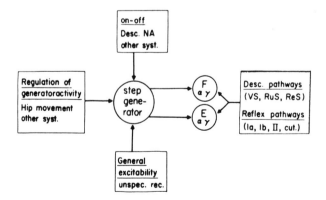

Figure 2 A speculative diagram of the circuitry involved in the generation of locomotion. (From Grillner, 1973.)

While the locomotion studies described above do not represent direct human evidence, the results of experiments on human locomotor patterns appear to confirm the presence, in normal man, of locomotor subroutines. Pal'tsev (1967), for example, utilized a method of monosynaptic reflex testing to identify changes in spinal motoneuron excitability that were spatially and temporally similar to a locomotor synergy. It is known too that a newborn baby exhibits primitive stepping behavior well before he or she has learned to walk (Zelazo et al., 1972).

Even if genetically determined subroutines do exist can they really be a part of learned, skilled, and complex motor acts and if so, how? Questions such as this must still remain in the minds of many because of the traditional and lingering notion of reflex patterns being rigid, fixed, and invariant motor responses. The next section reviews evidence suggesting to the contrary: that reflex motor patterns themselves are modifiable and can be conditioned in exactly the same way as the rudiments of voluntary movement are thought to be conditioned in the acquisition of certain complex motor skills.

2. Subroutine Conditioning and Plasticity

In 1905, Twitmeyer reported the results of a study on normal males in which he demonstrated that the patellar reflex could be conditioned to the sound of a bell. Over a series of some 105–238 trials, a bell was rung 0.5 sec prior to percussion of the patellar tendon. At the end of the series, when the bell was sounded but no tendon tap delivered, a completely recognizable knee jerk was forthcoming. The significance of this finding was missed by the psychologists of the day and indeed for over 70 years little mention was made of the demonstration (Twitmeyer, 1974).[2] The fact that reflexes (subroutines?) can be elicited from a central source after a suitable period of conditioning fits perfectly with Easton's hypothesis of the reflex pattern composition of volitional movement (cf. Figure 1), for it demonstrates that the spinal reflex patterns are accessible to higher motor control centers. It further suggests that a reflex pattern conditioning process could serve as the base for the learning of certain motor skills, a process already described by some as the "reflexization of movement" (Asami, 1971). What would appear to be conditioned, however, is a "trigger or set of triggers" capable of evoking the reflex patterns. This set has been described elsewhere as an "algorithm of reflexes" (Marteniuk and Hayes, 1975).

In addition to their susceptibility to conditioning, man's reflex patterns are sufficiently plastic to enable adjustments and refinements to be introduced depending on the context in which they are to be used. Work by Hagbarth and

---

[2] See Twitmeyer (1974) for a discussion of the dissertation and, in particular, for the editorial comment by D. Grant.

Kugelberg and their colleagues has shown that man's abdominal skin reflexes and responses to painful stimuli possess a degree of functional adaptability, which implies a type of learning in some of the supposedly most stable pathways of the neuraxis (Hagbarth, 1960; Hagbarth and Kugelberg, 1958; Hagbarth and Finer, 1963). Similar observations of adaptability in reflexes have been made in a variety of other experimental situations. Melvill Jones and Watt (1971) have interpreted the second burst of electromyographic activity in human forearm muscles during rapidly imposed stretch (Hammond, 1954; Hammond *et al.*, 1956) as a supraspinal "functional stretch reflex," which is readily modified by prior instructions to the subject. Thus, when the subject was told to resist the stretching of his muscle, the observed reflex response was large, whereas following instructions to release or "let go," the reflex activity was very much diminished (Hammond, 1954, 1956; see also Newsom Davis and Sears, 1970). Our own results obtained from the deltoid muscle have confirmed this phenomenon (Hayes *et al.*, 1974).

Evarts (1973; Evarts and Tanji, 1974) has interpreted this effect of the "set" of the subject in terms of "gating of cortical reflexes." He states with respect to monkeys, ". . . although the short latency of the 30 to 40 msec EMG response suggests that it is a reflex, its acquisition through learning and its sensitivity to 'set' are features usually attributed to voluntary movement [Evarts, 1973]." The analogous situation in human kinesthetic reaction time studies employing joint displacement as the stimulus has not gone unnoticed (Hayes and McMillan, 1974; Hayes *et al.*, 1974). The analogy supports the notion of supraspinal "long loop reflexes" (Phillips, 1969) forming a substrate upon which are built rapid kinesthetic reaction times.[3] Whether or not this hypothesis can explain the extremely short latency error corrections that have been reported (Gibbs, 1965; Hick, 1949; Higgins and Angel, 1970) remains to be seen.

Adjustments or modifications of the later components of reflexes, presumably involving long supraspinal pathways, are thus well documented. It is acknowledged, too, that adjustments of the sensitivity of spinal reflexes are part of the changes known to precede voluntary movements and are localized to the region of the intended action (Kots, 1969; Kots and Zhukov, 1973). More generalized changes in spinal reflex excitability may also be accomplished through muscle contraction in other body parts (Hayes, 1972) and changes in gain of the "gamma loop' most probably also play an important role in peripheral motor control (Marsden *et al.*, 1971). Without recourse to neurophysiological detail the concept of reflex plasticity has thus been introduced to dismiss the once held idea of reflex patterns being invariant and rigidly defined configurations.

The suggestive evidence in support of the notion of inherent (reflex patterns) and acquired (conditioned "triggers" for reflex patterns) subroutines does not

---

[3] This would appear to be a physiological analog of stimulus response compatibility.

describe how the "motive" to move is translated into the observed motion. Theories concerning this issue have been put forward by Greenwald (1970), Konorski (1967), and Marteniuk and Hayes (1975). All of these theories suggest that a motive is elaborated into some internal representation of the desired movement, or its outcome, and in conjunction with affective input and associations derived from prior experience (motor memory?) a sequence of motor commands (triggers and subroutine modulations?) is formulated. Once again, neurological analogs of these processes may be suggested and we might look to the limbic system for the "drive to move," to the frontal and parietal cortex for the needed associations, and to the cerebellum and basal ganglia for the organization of the motor response prior to activity in the motor cortex (Brooks, 1974).[4]

Thus far, consideration of task complexity from the preprogramming viewpoint has focused mainly upon neurological evidence. While continuing to look at preprogramming we now turn to the behavioral studies pertinent to task complexity.

B. The Memory Drum Model

In 1960, Henry and Rogers presented their memory drum model of motor control. They postulated the existence of nonconscious mechanisms in the brain that use stored information (motor memory) to channel already existing nervous impulses into the appropriate neuromotor coordination centers, subcenters, and efferent nerves, causing the desired movement. The memory drum analogy was proposed as an attempt to help explain the relationship between response complexity and reaction time and was specifically formulated with fast preprogrammed movements (no feedback) in mind. Specifically, the memory drum model postulated the storage of motor "programs" (analogous and herein referred to as "subroutines") that could be called upon when a movement was to be initiated and then organized into the desired temporal and spatial arrangement. No structuring of the subroutines per se was thus required in the central organization process.

One of the testable predictions from the memory drum concept was that there should be a longer reaction latency for a complicated movement than for a simpler movement. It was reasoned that a more comprehensive program would require more processing time for the neural impulses to become coordinated and directed into the eventual output channels. Experimental support for this hypothesis came from the Henry and Rogers study of subjects performing tasks

---

[4] The paper by Brooks (1974) approaches the question of the complexity of organization and control of movement from a different and illuminating perspective: viewing the programming process as a spectrum of complexity with goal setting at the highest level and the end result, for example, extension of the arm and grasping, as the lowest level.

which demanded rapid initiation and which varied in the complexity of the movement phase. As predicted, longer reaction times (RTs) were associated with more complex movements.

From their results, Henry and Rogers implied that movement complexity was a function of the demand for accuracy and involvement of feedback in the control of movement. More definitely they claimed that complicated movements necessarily involved several muscle groups in several specific areas of neuromotor coordination centers. These were the only indications of the "crucial elements" of movement complexity contained in the Henry and Rogers model. While somewhat vague in its specifications, the memory drum model has led to further research concerned with identifying the elements of complexity.

1. Movement Extent and Response Complexity

One presumed element of response complexity that has received considerable attention is that of movement extent. The prediction from the memory drum model would be that movement extent is an element of complexity and thus longer movements would be preceded by longer RTs. Even before the memory drum model had been formulated, Brown and Slater-Hammel (1949) had investigated the relationship between a movement's length and its reaction time. Based upon movement amplitudes of 2.5–40 cm they reported that choice RT was quite independent of the distance moved. It is worth noting here that these small amplitude movements were to a specified location; from the early work of Woodworth (1938) we know that RTs in this situation are noticeably longer than when the subject is merely required to release a telegraph key.

In 1971, Williams reported a brief study in which RTs for a large response (a forward, right-arm swing in the vertical plane to grasp a pull-out string) were contrasted with the RTs for small responses (key release) reported in other investigations (Harrison, 1960; Henry and Rogers, 1960). The hypothesis being tested was the memory drum prediction that large amplitude movements would be preceded by a long RT. Reaction time was indeed reported to be some 25 msec longer for the gross movement employed in Williams' study and this was viewed as corroborative evidence for the memory drum concept. A note of caution must be expressed over this interpretation, however, for the studies across which the comparisons were made varied in stimulus modality and it is well known that auditory stimuli evoke more rapidly initiated responses than do visual stimuli (Whiting, 1969; Woodworth and Schlosberg, 1963).

The apparent difference between the findings of Brown and Slater-Hammel (1949) and the evidence presented by Williams (1971) prompted further investigation. Utilizing the technique of fractionating RT into premotor and motor time components, Lagasse and Hayes (1973) reported that elbow flexion movements of varied extent (one releasing a key and the other continuing through a 90° arc) were not preceded by different RTs. Providing more rigorous evidence against the notion of more central processing time being required for large movements was the fact that premotor reaction times did not differ for the two tasks. Premotor time (PMT) is the time lag between stimulus appearance and the onset of electromyographic activity in the responding muscle group. PMT is thought to provide a more sensitive index of central processing delay than does a total reaction time which includes a time lag (20–60 msec) for generation of sufficient muscular tension to move the limb from its resting position. The study by Lagasse and Hayes adds to the finding of Brown and Slater-Hammel, for in the latter, two specified end points with different movement amplitude were contrasted, whereas in the Lagasse and Hayes study two unspecified end points varying in movement amplitude were contrasted. Both studies found RT to be independent of movement extent.

The question of movement extent as a component of complexity and response latency was also studied by Glencross (1972, 1973), who, in a series of choice RT investigations, reported that changing the distance moved (6–18 in.) seemed to have little or no influence upon the latency of an elbow flexion response. The change in movement amplitude appeared to be accommodated within the subprogram. Only when task complexity was significantly changed by the addition of "directional control" contraints did response latency become longer. A somewhat related finding was that RT was independent of the force of the response. Although it was hypothesized that the recruitment of additional motor units and increased firing frequency of those units activated would constitute an element of complexity, this was not demonstrated. Instead, the relatively minor reorganization of the effector process needed to overcome a resistance of 15 lb, as opposed to 2 lb, was brought about by simple "... amplification or gain control" with no associated increase in response latency.

2. Movement Reversals

Another aspect of task complexity that has been subject to experimental scrutiny is that of rapidly executed reversals in the direction of fast movements. The memory drum model would predict that reversal in the direction of movement is an element of complexity; therefore, movements requiring directional changes should be preceded by longer RTs. The tasks utilized in the Henry and Rogers (1960) series involved many directional changes; because they were associated with longer RTs they would be interpreted in terms of the model as having influenced the RT by requiring more subroutines and thereby increasing the processing time.

Evidence from Glencross (1973) indicates that this is not necessarily the case. When a single direction reversal was required in his elbow flexion task the RT was no longer than for a single direction movement. Assuming that the response was preprogrammed, i.e., its agonist and antagonist muscle activity were specified by the efferent command, the effect of demanding a reversal was thus rather similar to increasing the antagonist activity to such an extent as to reverse the direction of motion.

It has become evident from the literature pertaining to the memory drum model that the elements of response complexity still await identification. Fortunately, the recent work of Klapp *et al.* (1974) appears to have shed some light as to why the conventional memory drum approaches (which have concentrated largely on simple RTs) have not met with a great deal of success in this respect. They argue that the Henry and Rogers' hypothesis should more appropriately fit choice reaction time data, for in the simple RT paradigm the subject knows which response is required and he/she may undergo the processes assumed in the memory drum theory prior to onset of the stimulus. In effect the "programming" element of a response may only be measurable when the subject is called upon to select an appropriate response after the stimulus has been presented. A further implication from the work of Klapp *et al.* is that practice represents a confounding variable and one that has contributed to the inconsistency of results associated with simple RT-memory drum studies.

The issue of task complexity thus far has been dealt with exclusively in terms of preprogrammed responses. Such a limitation is not meant to deny the importance of feedback, either in the overall picture of task complexity, or as part of a regulatory or control feature influencing the running of a motor program that lasts for longer than 0.2 sec. What is apparent, however, is that the overall concept of preprogrammed responses is suited for analysis of the complexity of tasks requiring fast initiation and execution, but that when longer duration tasks are to be analyzed, another dimension of explanation might be more appropriate. This becomes especially evident when consideration is given to the simultaneous interaction of elements such as the precision, amplitude, and direction of discrete or continuous movements. Fortunately, complex interactions of this nature (and others) may be appropriately handled by the use of an "information processing" approach.

III. Information Processing and Complexity

Perceptual-motor skills may be conceptualized as the result of a series of central nervous system operations that determine the degree to which the resulting movement matches the particular environmental demand that was initially responsible for the planning and execution of the movement. From this framework perceptual-motor skills are seen as being dependent on central operations; that is, they are determined by the information processing activities within the perceptual, translation, and effector mechanisms (Welford, 1968). In this regard the activities of the central mechanisms are called information processing. Information, as it is used here, involves all available sensory input but in particular implies uncertainty; whenever something that is not perfectly predictable happens to a person he is said to have been presented with information. From this it follows that in perceptual-motor skills there are two major sources of information with which the central nervous system operations must be concerned. One source arises from uncertainty in the environment in which movement must be performed. The other source arises from feedback a performer receives from executing the task.

Viewing perceptual-motor performance as an information-processing activity has a number of advantages. First, it presents a way in which perceptual-motor skills can be analyzed into component parts. While these components are not independent of each other, in that their interactions produce a skilled perceptual-motor act, some skills are obviously more dependent on one type of mechanism than another. A second advantage to treating perceptual-motor skills in this way concerns the amenability of this conceptual approach to quantification. One of the biggest difficulties when attempting to define the complexity of a perceptual-motor skill is the lack of any rigorous method for measuring complexity. However, treating perceptual-motor acts as information-processing activities makes them quantifiable through the use of information theory. When this is done the complexity of a motor skill is defined in terms of how efficiently the human performer can process information. In this way complexity becomes a relative term since a highly practiced performer can perform a given skill much more efficiently than an individual who has not practiced the movement; in this sense the skill might be complex for the beginner and easy for the individual who has had considerable practice.

In studying the complexity of perceptual-motor skills from an information-processing dimension the main variable of interest is the time taken to process information. In this regard there are two general information-processing activities that must be considered. The first deals with reaction time, which is the time taken by the central nervous system to transform input information into an appropriate movement. The second concerns movement control or those information processes that take place between the initiation and termination of the movement.

A. Amount of Information and Reaction Time

It is a well-known fact (Whiting, 1969; Welford, 1968; Keele, 1973) that the major delay in RT is caused by the time required by the central mechanisms to process information rather than by such peripheral factors as sense-organ activation time, nerve-conduction time, and muscle-contraction time. Furthermore, RT has been shown to be very sensitive to the amount of input information where fast reactions are associated with low information inputs and long reactions are related to large information inputs. This is particularly true of the unpracticed individual whose performance is usually characterized by lengthy delays representing the RT required to process the great amounts of information present. Kay (1971) explains this by pointing out that performance at this level of learning is characterized by movements punctuated by relatively long time gaps necessitated by the performer's need to successively react to changing environmental conditions as well as the variable feedback he receives from his movements. With practice, however, the performer's movements appear to become continuous in nature and very rapid. At the same time RT to the same environmental situations appears to substantially decrease and sometimes is eliminated altogether when a performer can anticipate the occurrence of events relevant to his performance.

Complexity of perceptual-motor skills in these terms is thus a relative term used to describe how efficiently an individual can respond to a given situation. With practice, efficiency increases so that the complexity of a given skill decreases. This raises the issue of what factors determine whether a skill is complex or simple for any given individual. The view here is that if one analyzes performance, the complexity of a skill is in direct proportion to the amount of information or uncertainty with which a performer is presented. Practice is thus seen as reducing the amount of uncertainty leading to faster, more efficient, performance. From this viewpoint one might argue that the complexity of a skill can be defined as the amount of information that must be processed by the perceptual, translation, and effector processes.

There is little doubt that the amount of information presented to a performer significantly influences the operation of the perceptual and translation processes of performance. This can be seen by examining experiments which vary the amount of information by making perceptual discriminations more difficult, manipulating temporal uncertainty, and by manipulating the number of events as well as their probability.

In terms of perceptual discrimination two studies (Henmon, 1906; Crossman, 1955) serve to illustrate what happens to RT when different aspects of input information are difficult to discriminate. Henmon required his subjects to discriminate rapidly which of two straight lines, exposed on a screen, was the shorter by pressing one of two reaction keys. He found that the more the two lines came to resemble each other the longer the RT. Crossman found similar results when his subjects sorted specially made cards into bins according to the number of dots that appeared at random locations on each card. For example, in one condition he prepared six decks of cards with each deck containing an equal number of cards with the following numbers of dots: 10/1, 10/5, 12/8, 12/9, 10/8, 12/10. Furthermore, the average amount of uncertainty or information presented to the subject was obtained so that a subject's average RT could be compared to this variable. The average amount of information, which can be thought of as perceptual uncertainty, increased as the ratio between the dots decreased. His results indicated that as perceptual uncertainty increased, RT increased in a linear fashion. Thus, these studies indicated that the time of a decision process is greatly influenced by the discriminability of the input information. In this case discriminability can be regarded as one element of stimulus complexity which affects the time the central mechanisms take to make a decision.

Another form of input information complexity that has been shown to influence the time to make decisions is temporal uncertainty. Klemmer (1957) observed the effect this variable had on RT in two ways. First, he calculated the amount of uncertainty arising from the length of the foreperiod, with longer foreperiods representing greater uncertainty because of a performer's inability to judge accurately the passage of time. Second, he determined the uncertainty arising from the situation where different foreperiod lengths were randomly varied. His results indicated that as average amount of temporal uncertainty increased (measured in bits of information), RT increased linearly.

A third source of input uncertainty in many perceptual-motor skills that can be present even when stimuli are readily discriminable and temporal uncertainty is at a minimum is that due to event uncertainty. In this respect, uncertainty can be manipulated by increasing the number of possible events in a reaction time situation (i.e., the choice RT) or by varying the probabilities of occurrence of several possible events. In this situation the amount of average information presented to a subject would increase as the number of possible events increased (assuming that all events are equally probable) or the probability of the occurrence of any given event was decreased. A third related manipulation of events in a choice RT experiment concerns the establishing of sequential dependencies among successive events. To the extent that a given event allows prediction of following events the average amount of information conveyed by the total number of events is reduced.

How do the above manipulations of information influence decision times? Hyman (1953) answered this question when he systematically varied the amount of information presented to a subject in a choice RT task in each of these three ways. His results unequivocally supported the view that RT is determined primarily by the amount of input information and not by the method by which it is manipulated. He showed that a linear function described the relationship between RT and amount of information, where longer RTs were associated with large amounts of information, regardless of how the amount of information was varied. Thus, as was the case when amount of information was varied by making stimuli less discriminable and by manipulating temporal uncertainty, the complexity of the task, as evidenced by longer decision times, was a direct function of the amount of information presented to a subject.

Another source of uncertainty related to decision time, but which is not amenable to measurement in terms of amount of information, concerns the processing of information in regard to the organization of the effector units or neural impulses required for movement execution. This process is what Glencross (1973) has likened to a compiler or assembler function. Evidence has been presented earlier showing that in some cases RT can be significantly influenced by this assembling process (Klapp *et al.*, 1974) but the difficulty has been in determining the elements that comprise the motor commands. One would suppose that if these elements can be defined, the amount of information confronting a performer when attempting to assemble a particular program would be the number of alternative elements available for the desired movements. The greater the number of possible elements available the more uncertainty a performer would be faced with in terms of selecting an appropriate class of elements for assembling into a motor program. Therefore, it would be expected that the complexity of a particular movement, in terms of the effector component of the total decision process, would be directly proportional to the total number of possible elements that could be included in a given motor program. The more complex a task, the longer it will take an individual to decide upon the right class of elements that should be incorporated into the motor program.

B. Amount of Information, Practice, and S-R Compatibility

As mentioned previously, a characteristic of highly skilled performers is that their decision processes do not appear to be influenced by the amount of information with which they are presented. What once involved complicated, time-consuming decision processes appears to be reduced to simple, almost automatic decisions. Experimental studies showing an increase in the speed with which decisions are made are of two types: those studies that allow subjects to practice a decision task over a relatively long period of time, and those studies that keep information content constant but manipulate the stimulus-response relationships of the experimental task.

Mowbry and Rhoades (1959) studied how practice influenced responses on a two- and four-choice RT appratus. After 42,000 trials of practice had been given, performance in the four-choice condition improved to such an extent over the improvement that occurred in the two-choice condition that decision times in the two conditions were equal even though the two choice condition had initially resulted in a substantially faster decision time. Evidently practice served to overcome the difference in the amount of information initially represented in these two conditions. Another study (Davis *et al.*, 1961), while not finding the same dramatic effect that Mowbry and Rhoades did, found that the rise of RT with degree of choice was markedly reduced.

Another factor responsible for decreasing decision times concerns the degree of relationship between stimuli and responses or, in other words, the degree of stimulus-response compatibility. Compatible relationships are those relationships which the majority of people believe to be the most natural. S-R compatibility becomes important when one considers the relationship between amount of information and decision time for a number of different tasks. As previously mentioned there is a positive linear relationship between these two variables, indicating an increasing decision time with increasing amount of information. However, some investigators (Fitts and Seeger, 1953; Brainard *et al.*, 1962; Hellyer, 1963) show the importance of stimulus-response compatibility for decision times by noting that this variable greatly influences the slope of the line relating amount of information to decision time. In cases where stimulus-response compatibility is low the slope is steep and where compatibility is high the slope is near zero. The most notable study showing this effect was one by Leonard (1959), who showed that by having vibration to the fingers as stimuli with the required response of pressing the vibrator when it came on, decision times to two, four, and eight alternative stimuli were essentially equal. Thus, in this case, when S-R compatibility was very high, the number of alternative events failed to have an influence on decision time.

Undoubtedly practice influences S-R compatibility in that the more practiced a task is the more likely the stimuli are seen as being closely related to the appropriate response. As Welford (1968) suggests, the connections between stimuli and their corresponding responses become "built-in" and thus are ready for immediate use. This saves the time usually necessary to associate a particular stimulus with its appropriate response, as occurs in unskilled performance, thus accounting for a considerable reduction in decision time.

Since it is difficult to carry out laboratory experiments on the influence that long-term practice has on decisions in perceptual-motor skills, the exact effects that result from prolonged practice are not known with any certainty. S-R compatibility is obviously one factor that reduces the complexity of the decision process through practice. Another factor, more on the input side of the decision process, has to do with selective attention. As Marteniuk (1975) has pointed out, the inexperienced performer must consider information from the environment that the skilled performer has ruled out of consideration because of his past experience. He can selectively attend to the information that is most relevant to his performance. Related to this of course is his ability to predict what event from a number of possible events will occur and when this event will occur. Furthermore, the skilled individual is able to recognize and take advantage of sequential dependencies among events which enables him to deal with "chunks" of information rather then with each individual event separately.

Some of the same factors that reduce the amount of input information for the decision process also serve to reduce the complexity of the output or effector side. Practice would presumably reduce the total number of motor elements seen as being appropriate for a given skill. Moreover, some motor elements might be prepared in advance because they are contextually more probable than others. Finally, sequences of motor elements can be built up that represent "chunks" or units of motor elements that are dealt with as a whole rather than as individual elements, thus considerably reducing their information load.

In summary, the main purpose of this section has been, first, to define complexity of a perceptual-motor act in terms of the amount of information that had to be processed by the central mechanisms responsible for organizing and initiating a movement and, second, to show that complexity must be considered a relative term because of the changes that take place in information processing through practice. In terms of the information load placed on the central mechanisms, an inexperienced performer, because he must consider many possibilities, must process a great deal of information to arrive at the point of movement initiation. An experienced performer, on the other hand, is required to process much less information from the same skill and as a result his decision processes are facilitated.

By applying an information-processing approach to the decision aspect of perceptual-motor skills it was also seen that the complexity of a decision is a function of several interrelated central mechanisms. For instance, one can speak of complexity in terms of the perceptual demands placed on the performer when he must discriminate signals that are similar in nature. Similarly, complexity may also arise from uncertainty concerning what signal from a number of possible signals will actually occur. Finally, it has been pointed out that uncertainty can also arise on the effector side of the decision process where there are a large number of possible motor elements that must be organized and initiated to produce a desired movement. Thus, not only is complexity of decision relative to the practice state of an individual but complexity may result from any one of several sources within the chain of events that eventually lead to movement initiation.

C. Amount of Information and Movement Control

To this point in the treatment of perceptual-motor skill complexity only those factors that influence the organization and initiation of movement have been discussed. We now turn to the problem of applying an information-processing approach to the quantification of the complexity of movement control. For ease of presentation, the decision processes that lead to movement initiation have been treated separately but this in no way implies that movement control is independent of the previously discussed central processes. In fact, it will be seen that movement control actually involves a series of central decisions, the number of which determines the speed of the movement.

The main purpose for treating movement control from an information-processing viewpoint is to equate the complexity of movement control with the amount of information a performer has to process in order to produce movements that are made with maximum speed and accuracy. As will be seen, the main variable that creates uncertainty in movement control is feedback; thus, for the purposes of this discussion, it is necessary to delimit discussion to those movements under closed-loop control. Presumably the control of open-loop movements, since by definition they do not involve processing of feedback during the execution phase, would not impose any information load on the performer after the closed-loop movement is initiated. Given this situation, the complexity of movement control can be seen as a function of two related factors. One would be the nature of the task and the information load it placed on the performer. The second would be the information load imposed on a performer by detecting and correcting movement errors during the execution of a movement. Related to this second factor would be the amount of information or uncertainty present in the feedback that a performer receives as he executes a movement. Information for the detection of errors would arise primarily from visual and proprioceptive feedback and the amount of information in such signals would depend on their degree of uncertainty. On the other hand, the complexity of organizing and initiating a movement for the purpose of nulling the detected error would be a function of the information processes discussed under the preceding section on decision time. In this way an observed error in movement would act as an input to the central decision mechanisms responsible for organizing and initiating movement.

1. Index of Difficulty

The first factor that must be considered when attempting to understand movement control complexity is the nature of the task a performer must undertake. For this purpose we turn to the work of Fitts (1954a) who used information theory to quantify the difficulty of movement tasks. Fitts reasoned that the difficulty of a movement was a function of two parameters: the amplitude of the movement and the required precision for terminating the movement. Using concepts derived from information theory he then formulated the index of difficulty (ID) which is

$$ID = \log_2 \frac{2A}{W} \text{ bits/response}$$

where A is the amplitude of the required movement and W represents the tolerance range for terminating the movement.

If the ID represents the difficulty or complexity of a movement task then one would expect that as the ID increased, movement time would also increase since the performer would have to process more information. This is in fact what Fitts (1954) and Fitts and Peterson (1964) found. By varying both required movement amplitude and the width of the target it was found that movement time linearly increased with increases in the ID. From their manipulations of movement amplitude and target width it was evident that movement time was dependent on both of these factors. If target width was held constant and amplitude increased, movement time increased and vice versa. Thus it appears that these two parameters specify quite accurately the complexity involved in moving a limb to a target.

An interesting feature of the results of the above two studies was the finding that RT was independent of the ID. In fact, RT was completely unaffected in that it remained constant over the entire range of task difficulties studied. This result at first glance seems surprising when contrasted to the results of the studies previously reviewed dealing with the relationship between complexity of preprogrammed responses and RT. Some evidence was presented earlier showing that increased task difficulty, defined from a motor program perspective, resulted in increased RTs. Perhaps the reason for the difference in outcome between these two sets of results can be accounted for by differences in experimental paradigms. In the studies examining motor program complexity the majority of movements were very rapid and open-loop in nature and as a result their parameters had to be specified before movement initiation. Complexity in this case is thus a function of information processes occurring before movement initiation. However, in the Fitts (1954) and Fitts and Peterson (1964) studies, only a small proportion of the movements studied could be considered to be preprogrammed (i.e., those movements whose total duration was less than approximately 200 msec), and the rest were of a duration which allowed feedback to be used in their control. For these two studies, movement times for the various IDs ranged from around 140 to over 700 msec. Thus the strategy of the subjects in these studies might well have been to initially only organize and initiate a movement designed to start their limb in the correct direction; after this was underway, process feedback for the purpose of correcting or modifying the movement in order that the target could be accurately obtained. In this way RT would be expected to be relatively constant over all levels of movement difficulty in that movement complexity is a function of the information processes that occur after movement initiation.

2. ID and Processing of Feedback

If, as the above literature on the ID suggests, the complexity of movement control is a function of movement amplitude and target width, what are the information processes that produce the relationship between the ID and movement time? As suggested previously, movement control complexity can be viewed as the information load imposed on a performer by the necessity to detect and correct errors of movement. One might expect that the more complex a task, as expressed by the ID, the greater the possibility of a performer making errors in this movement execution. To detect these errors a performer would have to use either visual or proprioceptive feedback and the research literature indicates that the minimum times necessary for processing these types of feedback is rapid enough to allow their use in movement corrections. For instance, Keele and Posner (1968) found the minimum time for use of visual feedback in movement control to be somewhere between 190 and 260 msec, while Chernikoff and Taylor (1952) found that it took only about 110–120 msec for subjects to react to kinesthetic feedback. Thus it appears that both types of feedback are capable of being used to correct movements of relatively short durations.

Using evidence like the above, Keele (1968, 1973) has postulated that the observed function relating the ID to movement time can be explained by considering the number of corrections involved in a movement of given complexity. Keele argues that as the complexity of a task increases, as measured by the ID, the number of movement corrections also increase. Furthermore, if each correction takes an approximately equal time, the total movement time would be the product of the number of corrections and the time for each correction. Thus movement control complexity, as measured by movement time, is a direct function of the number of movement corrections required when executing a movement. While viewing movement control complexity in this manner accounts for the reason why some movements take longer than others, it does not explain why a given movement increases in velocity and accuracy over practice. In this respect, as in the decision processes, it appears that practice has the effect of reducing the amount of information necessary for movement control, thus allowing the performer to move faster.

3. Practice, Processing of Feedback, and the ID

Thus far two factors have been identified as contributing to the complexity of control. One was the nature of the task in terms of the information load imposed on the performer by the variables of amplitude and target tolerance. The second factor concerned a performer's ability to detect and correct errors rapidly since this was seen as the information process primarily responsible for determining movement time. The third factor for consideration concerns the effect that practice has on reducing the amount of information faced by a performer while controlling his movements.

Kay (1962, 1970) describes the changes in the information processes of movement control due to practice quite well. First, he showed (Kay, 1962) that on a task similar to that of Fitts (1954), subjects could substantially increase their speed of movement over 30 days of practice. Initially, his subjects performed at an information transmission rate of about 10 to 12 bits per second, which agreed with the rate found by Fitts (1954). After 30 days of practice, however, some of his subjects achieved rates of well over 20 bits per second. Kay concluded that this was a rather remarkable increase over just 30 days of practice and predicted that for highly skilled performers, who spend years performing some industrial task or athletic skill, the rate of information transmission would be considerably higher.

The cause of this increase in information transmission rate, however, is not an increase in the performer's capacity to handle information. Rather, as Kay (1962) points out, it is because of a decrease in the amount of information presented to a performer by a task of a given ID. In other words the ID of the task remains constant over practice; what changes is the way in which the performer processes information arising from feedback received while performing the task. Kay (1962, 1971) believes that the performer speeds up his performance not because he is processing more information (i.e., uncertainty) per unit time but because he is processing more feedback whose uncertainty is less. Consider the case where a performer initially undertakes to perform an unfamiliar movement. In this case the movement is performed slowly so that feedback, arising from visual and proprioceptive sources, can be used to compare the ongoing movement with some external criteria defining the movement. Over practice, the performer learns a great deal about the task through these two sources of feedback; this results in two changes in his information processing concerning the control of that movement. First, the performer comes to be able to select response units (Glencross, 1973) or subroutines that have a high probability of meeting the demands of the task. Thus, the uncertainty of the task had been decreased on the decision side of performance. Second, and just as important, because of the performer's familiarity with the feedback, and because he can accurately select a desired movement, he can predict in advance what the feedback characteristics of an appropriate movement should be. If the movement is then executed as intended, the feedback from the movement is redundant and as a result carries no information load. In essence then, it is only those feedback signals that deviate from the expected signals that a performer must attend to for the purpose of correcting the movement. In this way it can be seen that the information-processing demand of the practiced task is reduced considerably and as a result the performer can speed up his movement.

Inherent in the above explanation is the notion that because the selection of the correct subroutines improves with practice, the performer not only has a reduced information flow from feedback, but also has fewer movement corrections to make because of the relative accuracy of the initially selected response subroutines. In terms of the function relating the ID with movement time this means that movement time for any given value of ID will become faster because there will be fewer movement corrections to make. Thus it would appear that practice not only lessens the attention demand of monitoring feedback because of redundancy effects, but it also leads to fewer movement corrections for any given movement.

If we leave the discrete type of movement task and consider more continuous types of movements the same information analysis can be applied. Early in the acquisition of continuous movements performance would be slow and intermittent because of the large information load imposed on the central mechanisms. Through practice the performer would reduce the uncertainty in the perceptual and translation stages of the decision stage of performance in a way similar to that described for discrete tasks. However, the effector side of the decision stage would be more open to the development of motor programs, which would result in sequences of subroutines being executed as a whole. Such a motor program could be executed in an open-loop fashion thus reducing the necessity of the performer to monitor, through feedback, each individual component of the movement as it is executed. In this regard, one would expect that the performer would monitor the entire motor program and if it was executed as planned and had the desired outcome, performance would continue through executing further motor programs. The feedback received from such continuous movement would be redundant and carry no information load. On the other hand, if a motor program was erroneous in some respect, feedback would take some information value and through processing it the performer might organize a second sequence of commands for the purpose of achieving his desired results.

The acquisition of the above type of continuous movement control was seen in a study by Pew (1966). The subject's task was to keep a spot of light on an oscilloscope centered on a line. The spot would, if unchecked, move across the oscilloscope, disappear, and then reappear on the other side. The subject could stop and reverse the action of the spot by pressing a key with his index finger. The spot would then start accelerating; if the subject wanted to keep it on the oscilloscope he would have to press a second key with his other index finger. By alternating finger presses, the subject could keep the spot centered on the line.

Pew's results indicated that early in practice there were very obvious irregularities in the timing of key presses by the subjects. Their responses were under closed-loop control in that they made one response, waited for feedback, attempted another response, and so on. Later in practice the subjects shifted to an open-loop type of control where they grouped together a series of responses and executed them as a whole. Since there were about eight button presses per second, feedback could not have been used for monitoring each individual response. Thus performance appeared to be under motor program control at least for some of the time. Corrections were made by the subject, as he was operating in open-loop control, by noting the spot gradually shift from the center line and then issuing a single correction to bring the spot back on target. At this point he would reinitiate open-loop control. It would appear from this, that performance was facilitated by grouping several responses together into a motor program which not only represented an increase in efficiency over closed-loop control, where each response was initiated separately, but also considerably reduced the information load due to processing feedback.

One final type of control Pew found in some of his subjects was a modulation type. Here, the subjects would be in open-loop control but instead of initiating a single correction when they noted the spot drifting off the center line, they would modulate or modify the sequence of responses so that over several responses the spot would slowly drift back toward the center line. Performance here was constantly under the control of motor programs with feedback used to modify them to meet the specific demands of the task.

Summarizing this section, an attempt has been made to define those information-processing variables that must be considered when dealing with the control of complex motor skills. It was seen that complexity was a function of the nature of the task as measured by the ID, which was dependent on movement amplitude and target tolerance. The ID affects movement control by making the performer move slower for high values of the ID. The reason for this effect was related to the number of movement corrections necessary for successfully completing a task. It was argued that the more complex a movement, the more probability there would be of a performer making errors of movement and as a result there would be more corrections. However, through practice a performer can considerably reduce the information load imposed on him in a task by selecting subroutines that are more appropriate to the task. This has a dual effect on his performance. First, it allows him to predict the feedback consequences of his movement and, if the movement is executed as planned, leads to feedback being redundant which, in turn, reduces the information load. Second, more accurate movements result in fewer movement corrections. Both these factors are responsible for increasing movement speed for a particular task over practice. Finally, it was pointed out that the information load which determines the complexity of the control process can be further reduced by the formation of motor programs.

IV. Summary

We have tried to shed some light on the many questions that arise when trying to understand the control processes involved in different forms of complex motor behavior. Using two different dimensions of explanation, the preprogramming approach and the information-processing model, a large amount of experimental evidence has been covered and has been interspersed with quite a liberal dosage of speculation. What has become evident is that the issue of task complexity demands more consideration than merely attempting to identify the elements of the effector processes that contribute to the complexity. Since all perceptual motor acts depend to a large extent on decisions by several central nervous system mechanisms (perceptual, translation, and effector mechanisms), equal consideration must be given to these processes. Having arrived at this point the limitation of the preprogramming and the information-processing approach per se becomes evident and the holistic viewpoint obtained by considering both dimensions appears justified.

From the programming perspective perhaps the most important issues to evolve were the speculated means by which the complexity of the control process is minimized. The availability of subroutines would certainly appear to contribute to an optimally functioning system; we have attempted to add support to the hypothesis of Easton (1972) that in fact it is the body's inherent reflex patterns that provide the coordinative structures, or building blocks, from which voluntary movement may be constructed. If this is the case, one might hypothesize also that the stored triggering, sequencing, weighting, and modulation of the primitive motor patterns are what is contained in "motor memory." Undoubtedly, with practice, the motor memory would be updated and refined and more details of the sequencing and weighting, etc., would become stored.

If one views the degree of cortical control, which is most probably related to the amount of feedback and attention demands of the movement, as the earliest means by which refinements in a task are introduced, and with successive practice ingrained, then the process of learning will be paralleled by a lessening of cortical demands, reduced attention demand, and increased automatization of the control process. In other words, the complexity of the task will be minimized by virtue of the diminished information load and the greater dependence upon the relatively autonomous subroutines. This may well occur with no apparent differences in the overt response, although it is perhaps more likely that reduced errors, smoother coordination, and reduced energy requirements will also be manifest in the learned performance.

The speculated role of the cortex in the initial refinement of tasks is not a new idea. Hutton (1972) has summarized his views by noting that ". . . in the early stages the cerebral cortex must be constantly aware of what is being performed by long feedback loops. As voluntary movements are developed with experience the controlling pathways become more dependent upon cerebellar interventions and control." Ito (1970) has also suggested that as the learning process progresses, the "large loop through the external world" is replaced by an internal one passing through the cerebellum. This would serve as a model of the combination of the spinal motor system, the external world, and the sensory pathways. The shift from cortical control to cerebellar control would appear to parallel the servo control to preprogramming change implicated from Pew's work (1966). The only control demands that appear needed at this stage are the triggering, refinement, and error corrections of the gross "approximations" that have been produced (Marteniuk and Hayes, 1975).

References

Arbib, M.A. (1972). "The Metaphorical Brain." Wiley (Interscience), New York.
Asami, T. (1971). *Bull. Inst. Sports Med.* 9, 31–42.

Bossom, J. (1974). *Brain Res.* **71**, 285–296.

Brainard, R.W., Irby, T.S., Fitts, P.M., and Alluisi, E.A. (1962). *J. Exp. Psychol.* **63**, 105–110.

Brooks, V.B. (1974). *Brain Res.* **71**, 299–308.

Brown, J.S., and Slater-Hammel, A.T. (1949). *J. Exp. Psychol.* **38**, 84–95.

Bryan, W.L., and Harter, N. (1899). *Psychol. Rev.* **6**, 345–375.

Chernikoff, R., and Taylor, F.W. (1952). *J. Exp. Psychol.* **43**, 1–8.

Crossman, E.R.F.W. (1955). *Quart. J. Exp. Psychol.* **7**, 176–195.

Davis, R., Moray, N., and Treisman, A. (1961). *Quart. J. Exp. Psychol.* **13**, 78–89.

Easton, T.A. (1972). *Amer. Sci.* **60**, 591–599.

Easton, T.A. (1975). *In* "Psychological Aspects and Physiological Correlates of Work and Fatigue" (E. Simonson, ed.). Thomas, Springfield, Illinois.

Evarts, E.V. (1973). *Science* **179**, 501–503.

Evarts, E.V., and Tanji, J. (1974). *Brain Res.* **71**, 479–494.

Fitts, P.M. (1954). *J. Exp. Psychol.* **47**, 381–391.

Fitts, P.M., and Peterson, J.R. (1964). *J. Exp. Psychol.* **67**, 103–112.

Fitts, P.M., and Seeger, C.M. (1953). *J. Exp. Psychol.* **46**, 199–210.

Fukuda, T. (1961). *Acta Oto-Laryngol., Suppl.* **161**, 1–52.

Gardner, E.E. (1968). *Quest* **12**, 1–25.

Gibbs, C.B. (1965). *Brit. J. Psychol.* **56**, 233–242.

Glencross, D.J. (1972). *J. Mot. Behav.* **4**, 251–256.

Glencross, D.J. (1973). *J. Mot. Behav.* **5**, 95–104.

Granit, R. (1970). "The Basis of Motor Control." Academic Press, New York.

Greene, P.H. (1971). Quarterly Report No. 29. Institute for Computer Research, University of Chicago, Chicago, Illinois.

Greenwald, A.G. (1970). *Psychol. Rev.* **77**, 73–99.

Grillner, S. (1973). *In* "Control of Posture and Locomotion" (R.E. Stein *et al.*, eds.), pp. 515–535. Plenum, New York.

Hagbarth, K.E. (1960). *J. Neurol., Neurosurg. Psychiat.* [N.S.] **23**, 222–227.

Hagbarth, K.E., and Finer, E.L. (1963). *In* "Brain Mechanisms" (G. Moruzzi, A. Fessard, and E.H. Jasper, eds.), Vol. 1, pp. 65–78. Elsevier, Amsterdam.

Hagbarth, K.E., and Kugelberg, E. (1958). *Brain Res.* **81**, 305–318.

Hammond, P.H. (1954). *J. Physiol. (London)* 23–25.

Hammond, P.H. (1956). *J. Physiol. (London)* **132**, 17–18.

Hammond, P.H., Merton, P.A., and Sutton, G.G. (1956). *Brit. Med. Bull.* **12**, 214–218.

Harrison, J.S. (1960). *Res. Quart.* **31**, 590–600.

Hayes, K.C. (1972). *J. Appl. Physiol.* **32**, 290–295.

Hayes, K.C., and McMillan, K. (1974). *Proc. 8th Annu. Meet. Can. Ass. Sports Sci.* (Abstr.), p. 19.

Hayes, K.C., McMillan, K., and Charron, R. (1974). *Pap., Can. Symp. Psycho-Mot. Learn. Sport Psychol., 6th, 1974* (Abstr.), p. 20.

Hellebrandt, F.A., Houtz, S.J., Partridge, M.J., and Walters, C.E. (1956). *Amer. J. Phys. Med.* **35**, 144–159.

Hellebrandt, F.A., Houtz, S.J., Krikorian, A.M., Partridge, M.J., and Waterland, J.C. (1962). *Amer. J. Phys. Med.* **41**, 56–66.

Hellyer, S. (1963). *J. Exp. Psychol.* **65**, 521–522.

Henmon, V.A.C. (1906). *Arch. Phil. Psychol. Sci. Methods* **8**.

Henry, F.M., and Rogers, D.E. (1960). *Res. Quart.* **31**, 448–458.

Hick, W.E. (1949). *Quart. J. Exp. Psychol.* **1**, 175–178.

Higgins, J.R., and Angel, F.W. (1970). *J. Exp. Psychol.* **84**, 412–416.

Hutton, R. (1972). *In* "The Psychomotor Domain: Movement Behavior" (R.N. Singer, ed.), Chapter 13. Lea & Febiger, Philadelphia, Pennsylvania.

Hyman, R. (1953). *J. Exp. Psychol.* **45**, 188–196.

Ito, M. (1970). *Int. J. Neurol.* **7**, 162– 176.

Kay, H. (1962). *In* "Defense Psychology" (A. Geldard, ed.), pp. 161–169. Macmillan, New York.

Kay, H. (1971). *In* "Mechanisms of Motor Skill Development" (K.J. Connolly, ed.), pp. 139–151. Academic Press, New York.

Keele, S.W. (1968). *Psychol. Bull.* **70**, 387–403.

Keele, S.W. (1973). "Attention and Human Performance." Goodyear, Pacific Palisades, California.

Keele, S.W., and Posner, M.I. (1968). *J. Exp. Psychol.* **77**, 155–158.

Kennedy, D. (1973). *In* "Control of Posture and Locomotion" (R.E. Stein *et al.*, eds.), pp. 428–436. Plenum, New York.

Klapp, S.T., Wyatt, E.P., and Mac Lingo, W. (1974). *J. Mot. Behav.* **6**, 263–271.

Klemmer, E.T. (1957). *J. Exp. Psychol.* **54**, 195–200.

Konorski, J. (1967). "Integrative Activity of the Brain." Univ. of Chicago Press, Chicago, Illinois.

Kots, Ya.M. (1969). *Biophysics (USSR)* **14**, 176–183.

Kots, Ya.M., and Zhukov, V.I. (1973). *Biofizika* **16**, 1085–1091.

Lagasse, P.P., and Hayes, K.C. (1973). *J. Mot. Behav.* **5**, 25–32.

Lashley, K. (1917). *Amer. J. Physiol.* **43**, 169–194.

Laszlo, J.I. (1966). *Quart. J. Exp. Psychol.* **18**, 1–8.

Laszlo, J.I., and Manning, L.C. (1970). *J. Mot. Behav.* **11**, 111–124.

Leonard, J.A. (1959). *Quart. J. Exp. Psychol.* **11**, 76–83.

Marsden, C.D., Merton, P.A., and Morton, H.B. (1971) *J. Physiol. (London)* **222**, 32–34.

Marteniuk, R.G. (1975). *In* "Readings in Human Performance" (H.T.A. Whiting, ed.), pp. 7–35. Lepus, London.

Marteniuk, R.G., and Hayes, K.C. (1975). *In* "Readings in Human Performance" (H.T.A. Whiting, ed.), pp. 119–139, Lepus, London.

Melvill Jones, G., and Watt, D.G.D. (1971). *J. Physiol. (London)* **219**, 709–727.

Mowbry, G.H., and Rhoades, M.V. (1959). *Quart. J. Exp. Psychol.* **11**, 16–23.

Newsom Davis, J., and Sears, T.A. (1970). *J. Physiol. (London)* **209**, 711–738.

O'Connell, A.L., and Gardner, E.E. (1972). "Understanding The Scientific Bases of Human Movement." Williams & Wilkins, Baltimore, Maryland.

Orlovsky, G.N. (1972). *Brain Res.* **40**, 359–371.

Pal'tsev, Ye.I. (1967). *Biophysics (USSR)* **12**, 1048–1059.

Pew, R.W. (1966). *J. Exp. Psychol.* **71**, 764–771.

Pew, R.W. (1974). *In* "Human Information Processing: Tutorials in Performance and Cognition" (B.H. Kantowitz, ed.), p. 1. Erlbaum, New York.

Phillips, C.G. (1969). *Proc. Roy. Soc.* **173**, 141–174.

Schmidt, R.A. (1975). *Psychol. Rev.* **(in press)**.

Shik, M.L., Severin, F.V., and Orlovsky, G.N. (1966). *Biophysics (USSR)* **11**, 756–765.

Taub, E., and Berman, A.J. (1963). *J. Comp. Physiol. Psychol.* **56**, 1012–1016.

Taub, E., Bacon, R., and Berman, A.J. (1965). *J. Comp. Physiol. Psychol.* **59**, 275–279.

Taub, E., Ellman, S.J., and Berman, A.J. (1966). *Science* **151**, 593–594.

Twitchell, T.E. (1971). *In* "Mechanisms of Skill Development" (K. Connolly, ed.), pp. 25–38. Academic Press, New York.

Twitmeyer, E.B. (1905). *Psychol. Bull.* **2**, 43–44.

Twitmeyer, E.B. (1974). *J. Exp. Psychol.* **103**, 1047–1066.

Welford, A.T. (1968). "Fundamentals of Skill." Methuen, London.

Whiting, H.T.A. (1969). "Acquiring Ball Skill, A Psychological Interpretation." Bell, London.

Williams, L.R.T. (1971). *N. Z. J. Health, Phys. Educ. Recreation* **4**, 46–52.

Woodworth, R.S. (1938). "Experimental Psychology." Holt, New York.

Woodworth, R.S., and Schlosberg, H. (1963). "Experimental Psychology." Methuen, London.

Zelazo, P.R., Zelazo, N.A., and Kolb, S. (1972). *Science* **176**, 314–315.

Index